The Talking Cure:
New and Selected Poems

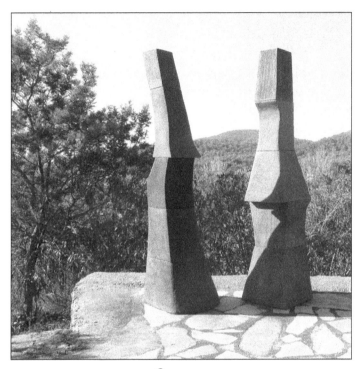

Jack Coulehan

Plain View Press, LLC
1101 W 34th Street, STE 404

www.plainviewpress.net
Austin, TX 78705

ISBN: 978-1-63210-078-8
ebook ISBN: 978-1-63210-079-5
Library of Congress Control Number: 2020934181

Cover photo by Jack Coulehan
Sculpture in photo by Lisa Cairns
Cover design by Pam Knight

We Find Healing In Existing Reality

Plain View Press is a 40-year-old issue-based literary publishing house. Our books result from artistic collaboration between writers, artists, and editors. Over the years we have become a far-flung community of humane and highly creative activists whose energies bring humanitarian enlightenment and hope to individuals and communities grappling with the major issues of our time—peace, justice, the environment, education and gender.

in memory of my parents,
Peg and Lee Coulehan,
with boundless gratitude

As wind moves and stone
endures, let us walk
in pilgrims' joy
and hold among our gifts
the early songs
that burst in pain,
came in wonder, rose
to laughter,
while we grew to find
communion
in our odd enduring hope.

Contents

from

The Knitted Glove

(1991)

Anatomy Lesson

When I move your body
from its storage drawer,
I brush my knuckles,
Ernest, on your three-days
growth of beard. Cheeks,
wet with formaldehyde,
prickle with cactus.
My eyes burn and blink
as if a wind of sand
blew through the room.

Bless me, Ernest,
for I cut your skin
to learn positions
and connections
of your parts — caves,
canyons, fissures, faults,
all of you. Show me.
Show me your flowers,
your minerals, the oil
of your spleen.

Do not mistake these tears.
These tears are not
for your bad luck
nor my indenture here,
but for all offenses
to the heart — yours, mine —
for the violence
of abomination.
Think of my tears as rain
staining your canyon walls,
filling your stream,
touching the blossoms.

Finches

Cages stacked three deep against the wall,
I sweep seed, surrounded by wings
stuttering, wings that awaken
a little skip or a twist behind my breastbone.
I pull and replace wet papers
that separate the layers of cages
and try to imagine a kitchen
without finches, without the smell
of sawdust, without acidic excretions,
still the warmest room in the house
where I dress, standing beside the stove,
nursing a Sanka, but silent.
A kitchen without one hundred twenty-two
society finches, siskins
and canaries. I try to imagine
the freedom to stand at my window
at six, and watch the neighbors' dogs
pacing their rounds in the snow, briskly,
or the freedom not to come home at night.
There are two cages at the other end of my table,
each with two birds. Every nook and cranny
is apportioned to finches. The counter is covered.
It was not always like this. There was the night I found
the first finch, the first songbird to join me
in the kitchen. I try to imagine the silence
broken by its first song, like a camp
awakening in the woods, a long way
from conventional music. More than a hundred
birds later, I stand in my overalls
ready for work. Ready to go.
It's no good these finches filling my kitchen,
the smell and clutter, the bags of seed,
the neighbors complaining. Too much is too much.
Each day I try to imagine
opening a cage, taking a pair of these finches —
concealed under my coat like small
exuberant breasts — and setting them free.

The Knitted Glove

You come into my office wearing a blue
knitted glove with a ribbon at the wrist.
You remove the glove slowly, painfully,
and dump out the contents, a worthless hand.
What a specimen! It looks much like a regular hand,
warm, pliable, soft, you can move the fingers.

If it's not one thing, it's another.
Last month the fire in your hips had you down
or up mincing across the room with a cane.
When I ask about the hips today, you pass it off
so I can't tell if only the pain
or the memory is gone. The knitted hand
is the long and short of it, pain doesn't exist
in the past any more than this morning does.

This thing, the name for your solitary days,
for the hips, the hand, for the walk of your eyes
away from mine, this thing is coyote, a trickster.
I want to call, "Come out, you son of a dog!"
and wrestle that name to the ground for you,
I want to take its neck between my hands.
But in this world, I don't know how to find
the bastard, so we sit. We talk about the pain.

Lake Effect

Wrapped in your chair
like a rummage sale,
you blink with wetness
at the snow
without the limbs
to wipe your face.

Where lake's wet wind
hits land's cold air,
it snows like this
all winter — wind up,
light down, pond iced,
and geese.

A ragged arrowhead
bursts through
and honks at you.
Hunched at the edge
of a snowbank,
you honk, too — your throat

spurts where the words
won't burst — at sheer
grayness that rolls
above bare branches.
Those geese honk back.

And your lips — I think
they are the coast
of this small pond.
Your face, white slopes
around the pond

where geese like saviors
land. Your eyes —
my friend, your eyes
are hot springs
that warm those geese
all winter.

Banana Bread

Today, after all these months,
you're on the phone again
about the bread you promised
after Easter. You have the right
rotten bunch of bananas.
Your legs are down a little,
though not from the water pill.
If I could drive to evening Mass
with you, you'd give it to me
warm. You'd call a taxi
but the way a driver looked
at you last week — at sixty-
seven yet! Men have only
the one thing on their minds
and you're still young. First time
you called you wouldn't pay
my bill — why should you? — all I do
is talk and give you pills.
Next time your legs were fat
as alabaster columns,
as cold as granite. The next call
you wondered what I think
of women running wild, what with
birth control. The evil one
is in us all. The last call
you said I'll have that loaf
of warm banana bread
for Christmas. February.
April. This time there you are,
your legs warm as two
light loaves, risen and powdered.

Good News

The first bad news is a spot on my lung
when all I came to the doctor for
was a leg that burnt like scalding water.

Then they find a hole in my spine,
right at the place my back kicked out
the day I jumped an aluminum ladder.

But no, my doctor looks at the wall
and says this black egg growing in my back
is not that, it's something new.

Today's scan shows a hole in my liver
and, strangely, though I'm still not sick,
my body begins to die.

There's Drano dripping in my vein
to scour the blood clot, and each new day
brings another test and more bad news.

Toward the back of the morning paper
are stories of love and reunion,
tales of miraculous cures.

A retired butcher finds a girl
he courted in Palermo, 1946,
and they dance all night in Niles, Ohio.

Good news. That's what I want to hear,
not the next painful step on the ladder,
to the next lower rung.

Good news! If I ever get out of here,
I'll rent a bowling alley
and we'll dance all night in Niles, Ohio.

Anniversary

for Peg Coulehan, 1914-1986

Three years after you walked upstairs,
took out your rosary beads, lay down
and died, my daughter shows me,

pointing to the window as she eats,
a fat cardinal hopping our back steps,
its belly puffed like the bourgeoisie.

Yet, the bird's ascent from step to step
is ballerina light, so elegant
I remember birds in their bones

are air where the rest of us are thickness.
My son, his backpack slung for school,
points out that birds are dinosaurs,

creatures that did not die out but rose.
Their cold bodies blanketed in ash
first shed thickness, then solidity,

and hopped, then flew, to another age.
That fat cardinal floats on cold dirt
near the base of an azalea bush,

while I think of you, shedding thick cells
that held you close to the ground
and your shrunken brain that failed,

becoming a buoyancy, a grace
I sometimes feel, like this morning
in the breakfast room, an air

that hops between two junipers
and rises — my daughter points again —
to moist black bones of an aging oak.

from

First Photographs Of Heaven

(1994)

"Spaceship Takes Photographs of Heaven"

Propped in bed
in your blue dressing gown,
a bruised spot on your chin
reddens
when you grind your teeth
and your left arm flips
(*thwop-thwop*)
like a slow propeller.
You hide that left hand
under the dinner tray
and try to keep it still,
try to cram it between your legs
until the tray slides and milk spills.
Its (*thwop-thwop*) is dampened
by your bedclothes
and bound by another hand
but your clumsy, incessant brain
has rolled out of its hangar.
The more you try, the faster
it goes. It's not embarrassed.
Its engines are warming,
papers fly, your *National Observer*
flutters   flies   there go
the first photographs of heaven
there go the white spheres
the two-headed boy
the woman who waited forty years
for   (*thwop-thwop*)   this is a taxi
this is not a simulation
this is a B-17 taking off
on its next-to-last mission

Poison

In an open box beside my chair
sit vials of poison and the jar
of cream I use to smear my scalp.
My son comes in to check me out,
afraid that I'll forget to take
my poison, but I won't forget.

For heart I take a white one once.
For bowels a scarlet ball at night.
And when I think too much in bed
I take a lavender-and-green.
To keep my heart from beating fast,
a poison pill that binds me up.
For blood, high blood, a red-and-white.
For blood, low blood, I take a brown.
To make the prostate work I take
an elephant tablet twice a week.
Once, I smear my scalp with cream
to keep the sores from coming back.

My son brings my seven refills in
and asks if I would like some air.
It's warm, he says. *Let's get some rays.*
That boy sees poison in my eyes,
the poison working through my skin.
He wants to hold my hand, but he's
afraid. That makes two of us.
For heart I take a white one once.

The Man with a Hole in His Face

He has the lower part,
a crescent of face
on the right, and an eye

that sits precipitously
beside the moist hole
where the rest of his face was.

The hole is stuffed
with curls of gauze.

His nurse comes before dawn,
at the moment
the eye fears for its balance,

and fills the wound,
sculpting a tortured landscape
of pack ice.

The man's eye does not close
because any blink
is death,

nor does the eye rest
in mine
when I ask the questions
he is weary of answering.

While I wait here quietly
in artic waste,
the pack ice cracks
with terrifying songs.

Over the moist hole
where the rest of his face was,
he rises.

The Act of Love

How foolish Celia must look
to the Haitian cab driver
on the Medicaid run!

She wears a white communion dress
the week before Easter, a sign
she brings me something more pressing

than the pain in her shoulder
and the son who doesn't talk to her
because his wife is embarrassed.

Her hips creak in conversation,
her knees grind, but even crepitant joints
are modestly silent and stand aside

when Celia hands me a potted plant
for my office — *an act of Christian love*,
she says, *not a sign of being personal.*

As for me, I'm stunned
out of the ordinary anger
at failing to help her

by the waxy leaves of her gesture
and I receive this wafer of the season,
heartbroken for no reason.

Complications

The last time Nate came in
he smelled like Grace did when
she worked door-to-door
for Avon. He had the one
pierced earring in, his beard
was trimmed, he had the cane
with a devil's head, the one
Grace used to clobber him
the night she stroked. The last time
Nate came in, the housing cops
had been — they took his two
big dogs. And then he was
alone. No matter what he did
the kids would bust his locks
and trash the place.

Nate found a woman half his age
or she found him. He wound up
in Baltimore, drunk, without
a bank account and by himself.
When he made it home
both guns were gone. Then Nate
was put in jail for D & D
a time or two. At the end
they phoned me from the morgue —
in his pants the boys had found
an old appointment card and Nate's
Certificate of Satisfactory Service,
nothing else. They asked
if I would sign him out
and save the boys a trip?
I said, sure, *Let's give the man
a heart attack.* Then I thought
of Grace's stroke, only I
didn't say a word about Grace,
just, *Boys, the cause of death
was complications.*

McGonigle's Foot

Philadelphia, 1862

McGonigle is dense in thought,
a step beyond his bout with drink.
Filbert Street trips up his back
and turns his ankle from behind.

A foreigner, a drunk, and loud,
the surgeon scratches in his book.
No need to etherize this case.
That night they amputate the foot.

McGonigle is pinned to bed
by rippling arms, his swollen leg
is roped to frame. The surgeon saws
as quick as sex. The leg kerplunks.

Retching, terrified, and screaming,
the Irishman curses the Virgin
and Jesus. *Keep your distance, men,*
the surgeon in his apron warns.

The lower orders of the race
have nerves more coarse than ours,
a boon in light of all the shame
and filth unfortunates endure.

You must use ether wisely, men,
by judging risk against the gain.
The young men shift from foot to foot.
McGonigle goes down for good.

For pain is our Creator's gift
to teach and strengthen us, a most
desirable – though never sought –
companion, men. So, humbly, cut.

Alabama

In the ward
behind a curtain
with a sleeping cap
akimbo on her wig,
Alabama whispers
like a locomotive,
Let me go.

In some brown place
above her bed,
my stern professor stands
and frowns
at my attempts
to stoke the boiler
in her chest.

Wrinkled and abused,
this Alabama lies
in some deep structure
of my mind
where still I kneel
beside her freckled arms
pumping morphine, merc
and oxygen.

The distant locomotive chugs.
I slap her, *Dammit,*
Live

The Rule of Thirds

Third, third, third – the rule I learned
about the stories of the ill.

A third get well – joints begin to move,
pain improves, depression's dull

embrace is eased. The villain leaves
without a trace and no one knows

the hero's name – doctor
or patient, science or grace.

A third grow crippled in the pain
of joints gone stone, their minds decline,

the villain takes the loot no matter what
your dour professor does, or you –

in the arrogance of youth – might try.
We learn by progress in our minds.

A third remain the same. They take
the villain in, they harbor him

until his tale is theirs and theirs is his.
They visualize their bodies with his eyes.

Our rule of thirds was not as kind
as love's compassion is,

nor as thunderous as an essay
on machines, but it spoke

the language of the body
in its genes.

My Father Sends Me Out for Tobacco

My father, the Lebanese coach,
sends me out for tobacco
while the other guys take gym.
It's roundball, B-ball, hoops, a knot
of legs and filthy skinny shirts
slamming down the court September,
April, May. In America
soccer has yet to be invented.
Tennis is the fairy's sport. The sons
of miners work at football
for redemption. Their skinny brothers
play the hoops for Lash, my father.
He spits into his can and swears and paces,
a small, dark figure
across the cavernous gym —
foul, unshaven. Players know
my father's rage will strike them
sometimes without warning,
will throw them against their lockers
and hit unjustly where it hurts.
My father saves me from insults
by saying not to suit up.
Get me some Mail Pouch
and get your ass back here
to pick up this equipment.
I hear those hollow whips of sound
and see the fearsome sweat
of boys aching for Lash. I see
the bleachers folded like sarcophagi.
I feel the emptiness. The rage
of my father, the Lebanese coach,
fills about half of the emptiness.

Tumbleweed

Took him 28 years
to pick up
that pack of cigarettes.

One night my father re-appears
in a phlegmy voice
from Sunny Farms in California.

When I arrive, he's on the porch,
his fingers
in a plastic cup of juice.

Working white restraints around his chest,
my mummy of Houdini
whispers, *Guess your momma bit the dust.*

He shows a box of photographs.
Lookee here.
There's Fairbanks, Heston, Gable, Leigh.

He says he worked a hundred flicks,
played bit, walked on,
marched for Caesar, fought Napoleon.

You haven't changed a bit, he says.
I was eleven when he left.
You musta seen me ride beside the Duke.

In swirls of dust, a thousand steer
stream below vermilion sky
while cowboys disappear.

My father wipes the drool into his cup,
A loner's like a tumbleweed,
he breaks off, blows away, dries up.

The Dust of the West

My blind father loves to stir the dust
of the West and kick the mare's flanks.
He cannot see the dazzling leather boots
he wears are covered with silky dust,
nor can he see the crust of dull sand
on his Levis. Blind and wild, he rides
out of Greasewood, whooping and hollering.
Behind his old saddle, my father carries
the camera that Edward Curtiss carried
and the tripod and hood that Curtiss used
when he shot the soul of the West.
A wind shakes and tosses the ochre dust
that clings like a cloud of bees to his back.
He is blind as a bat, obsessed with the thought
that specks of the desert are alive.
The smallest piece of dust has an interior,
a soul different from the souls of animals.
Still, an *inside* that strives to restore itself,
surrounded by a palpable light
that pours through my father's skin
as the sun rushes through a person's eyes.
By sensuously perceiving the dust
as it sits undisturbed on the surface
of things, by capturing whatever he finds
suspended in the sepia landscapes
that Curtiss created, my blind father
believes he can burst open the dust
and release its exquisite kernel —
the blessings of dirt, gathering and rising.

Jerusalem

My black father touches a poinsettia bush
on his morning walk, and from the back
he looks like a praying mantis. He walks out
to greet the iceman, the sun of Jamaica.
My father asks for a little more time
to answer my questions, to give me
the words I need. He pleads for patience.
We drive through pits between the hills
to see a hundred sick at clinic.
They cry for the belly, they toss at night,
their skin prickles with jaundice,
their sores will not heal. My father
fills their empty Kola Champagne bottles
with tart, black medicine. He delivers
a thousand from death by putting a knife
to their bodies, a thousand from death
by spraying the swamps for mosquitos,
a thousand from death by preaching the Bible.
The Queen receives him in London
and gives him the Empire. My father
puts the British Empire into a drawer
of memories. We listen to hymns in the dark.
We listen to fierce cries of Jamaica
so compelling that crabs lumber toward them.
My father takes me to Kingston, a city
smoldering under the weight of tin and grease.
He eats vegetables, plantain, and Postum.
I take peppered crayfish and chicken.
My father asks for a little more time.
He begs me some patience for the future.
Later, when I see him swollen
like an old tree dying of fungus,
still, he brings me visions of Jerusalem,
a black city full of his sons.

Labrador

When the universe ages
only a cold grey soup of matter
will blow endlessly forward
from the beginning. Today that soup
roars and pitches the ferry
across Belle Isle Strait.

Outside the cabin, I look toward the Labrador coast
where chunks of the continent still hold on.
I squint in molecular rain.
Puffins dive and skid with the vengeance of protons
in an accelerator, ripped apart
and burst into the angular traces of time,
that most ambiguous direction.

Inside the cabin, truckers finish their eggs
and wipe their plates with the last
pieces of toast. The cook sizzles some chunks
of butter on the grill. Labrador moans
outside on the strait. Cod fishermen's horns
burrow into the wind. This music is never heard

in the south, only the hoarse threat of music
reaches down to the conifer forest;
farther south, nothing. The cabin door
swings open one moment; swings closed the next.
Slam open! Two women play cards at the bar,
salmon fishermen snooze. Slam closed! Magnetic north

draws the unconnected molecules of everything
into Labrador. I see thoughts I had neglected
to pin down spin wildly, flying north.
I see parts of my body tumble into wind and disappear.
My vision of Labrador
dives like a predatory bird and soars.

St. Ronan's Finger

Inishmore, Galway

Because the south-south-westerly wind
arrives with evening, the island is swept clean
down to huts the size of stone ovens, down
to a bone in the shrine of St. Ronan,
to a cross so ancient that what remains of it
is a limestone phallus. Swept clean down
to walls and walled paths, to a hoary iron bell
marked with a cairn. Because wind torments
the cliffs of this island and lashes
its limestone fissures, and the fissures are filled
with delicate fronds, small ferns, ledge moss,
legends, coarse sand, crowns of thorns, and echoes
of monks, I am swept clean.

Because my eyes squint in the wind, I see
St. Ronan lugging wooden buckets of seaweed
up a treacherous path from the coast
and dumping them in gullies between rocks.
St. Ronan is creating soil, creating
a future for Inishmore from fucus and kclp,
souls and skeletons, bucket by bucket, year
by year. Now, because evening is rushing in,
I feel St. Ronan's finger's almost
leaf-like tremor touching my chest
at its softest point, the arrow point.

My Uganda

for Sister Concepta Najjemba

Sister scans the hills
for burning weeds —
whatever she sees
is Uganda.

She sips lemonade
on the porch steps,
watches the roofs
for menacing birds
and suffers sleeplessness —
sleep is Uganda.

Sister's pale blue habit
is a vista so distant
that barefooted runners
carry tales
across her savannah.

Enveloped by the spoor
of Africa, she sways
and tells tales
of midnight raids
and dead cattle,

her father
shackled to a chair
as they shock him
in the balls,

her brother
necklaced to a tire,
doused with gasoline
and set afire.

When sister speaks
about the tragic fever
that carries her country
out of its senses, her body is
Uganda

While the other sisters
sleep, Uganda sits
at the edge of her bed.

She runs her hands
along her thighs,
she whispers *mai mai*
softer
than the vibrating fan.

Sister's fingers
ripple through the dark.
Her prayer
is medicine, her prayer
is sweet,
sweet medicine.

Lima Bean

I have carried this lima bean
since Holy Week, a year ago.
In my pocket the bean has not softened
nor sprouted. It is still
small, smooth and utterly different.
Like tops of monastery pews
its curvature is pleasing.

This lima bean is alive.
A faint disappearance
of nutrients, week after week,
continues. When I touch the bean
I am probing a deep pocket.
Inside the stony fibers
something still is carried forward.

from

The Heavenly Ladder

(2001)

The Window of My Discontent

At the base of the window above my desk
the screen has pulled from its frame
where fat-bodied insects once squeezed in
only to die in their prison.

Six of them — dark, dried shapes
dotting the space between windows,
pasted against a skim of debris —
grime and straw — the strokes of a mad calligrapher.

You simply cannot escape the way
your imagination works.
Chekhov once informed his friends that his next
project was the great novel —

no more small stuff, no more tales and sketches.
He intended to capture the deep nuance of mystery
and reveal its structure.
So he went to the country and listened.

He paid attention to the speech of the constable.
He listened to the horse thief talk.
He experienced the pain of a desperate woman
after her lover went home — a handful of lies,

a few inexplicable truths. This moment
is the only moment I have.
How can I give form to the passion that burns
in my stomach? How can I open up, give voice,

turn these words into flesh? Nothing can restore
those chips of life, nor understand
the helter-skelter strokes of dried straw.
This, too, is the beginning of my tale.

D-Day, 1994

Your arm is gone
to cancer at 30 — no honor
in that. The potato-like stump
is not where the pain is.

You take your pills
and watch TV —
where beaches in France
swim with images of old men
pacing the coast for the first time
since going down.

You notice their limps
and imagine the vacancies —
fear, lost limbs, their buddies dead.
Who would have thought
that first tide of grunts
attacking that fortified coast
could win the war?

You ask if a scan would explain
the pain in your phantom limb,
believing a scan is like a story
that reveals things. Those men
creeping the grey-crossed breast
of a hill on the coast of France —
they know what they lost, they know
what they are looking for.

The scan will not give you an answer.
You are looking in the wrong place
for an answer. The world works hard
to hide its D-day —
deception, danger, death,
deliverance. I wish I could give you
the old men's stories. I wish I could give you
their battles, which are almost used up
but still true.

Soundings: Three for the Stethoscope

1.

Let me place
these miniature pears
in my ears, this diaphragm
against your skin.

Listen — the wafting
of a cracked Victrola's voice
in the leaves of your garden.

2.

Wafting? What a word
for a simple
sonic phenomenon.

Leaves? I better stick
to the facts.
The noise is turbulence.

Garden? From plastic tubes
around my neck
a bell-shaped tuber.

3.

I slide the tuber
to the curve of your breast —

in an age of perfect machines,
how impertinent
to choose imperfect means! —

a waft of thuds and turbulence
instead of blips,
the scratch of tissue, this.

The Doctor's Wife

Years later she came to me
for a menagerie of shots
and some advice on water
in New Guinea. It didn't take
a minute to notice the tic
that had sprung up since the last
bout of whatever her illness was
and the devastated nails.
Her church was sending her
for three months, maybe six,
to a site on the north coast
where thousands of refugees
had fled to escape a war
on the next island, a conflict
that hadn't made the news
so far. They needed a nurse
more than a preacher, but she
volunteered for both. I wished
we had more time to talk
that morning. Her waxen aura
was singular, like speaking
to a statue by candlelight.
It's hard to explain. The Church
was sending a team with her,
plus some outdated medicines
from the clinic. She withdrew
her eyes from my desk at last
and whispered, *He always wished
to do God's work in the missions,
didn't he?* I had never met
the man. He placed that bullet
in his head before I came
to town. I knew the handwriting
that he used to cure the sick, though,
and the once-vivid stories
of his compassion. *He's looking
over your shoulder in this,*
I said. *Remember that.*

Isn't

Let me see if I have this right
about what it isn't. It isn't
the sugar. It isn't the blood clot.
It isn't you're just not telling me
because you think I'm too far gone
and can't handle it. And mostly
it isn't what I think it is.

I say my kidney feels like a bad
punch, but you say, *No, it isn't
the kidney. The kidney's the champ
of your body.* I say my knees
buckle, my head reels, and you say,
*Take one to keep calm and some
aspirin, but not on an empty
stomach. For God's sake, relax.*

What you mean is — *Get out!
I don't care about you. I don't
need you.* But the monster
comes craning its popped eyes
at everyone sooner or later,
even you. So relax. I hope
when you feel its sour breath
at your back, I'll be there to say
there's nothing to fear, it isn't
the monster. And anyway, it's
too early to know. Come back
when it's bigger.

Scents

Antiseptics sweeten, but cannot disguise
a deep intensity of urine in the home
where Justin Daly lives. Accidents pile up
on every shift — bags leak, sheets soil, shit smears.
An aide crams an armful of soaked clothes
into a canvas bin and swabs the floor,
but Justin, a bald man strapped to his seat,
pays no attention. He savors the scent
of the newly macadamized road
in Southfield, Jamaica, beside the graveyard
of the Seventh Day Adventist Church,
where his wife, or maybe his daughter, is buried.
Pimento. Hibiscus. He delights in the smell
of savannah dripping with rain; forbidden perfume.

Natural History

About survival the trees of Australia
have it right — keep up. Don't waste moisture
on beauty. Don't worry about the next
engaging bloke who wants to be inspired
by the landscape. Don't cream your face
to find pleasure, but hunker into the cracks
for the long haul. Thicken your leaves
to lessen the surface. Polish them
tight and hard like fried chips. If you need to,
strangle the life from a few of your limbs
until they whiten and drop. The maroon stain
of sap you splay across the tortured trunk
of your body is not the calamity
you imagine. Regarding survival,
ugliness is a blessing. That which stands
alone, fits in. Dead limbs make good trees.

Barnacles

After five years mulling about finches
and tortoises, he knew that perfection
was a product of chance. What next, he asked?
It wasn't long before the sickness came
and forced him to slow down. Who could he trust
with the manuscript? How much suffering
would it cause? Emma was already terrified
about the direction his soul would take
after death. The months of work this sickness
would chew-up were a small price to pay
for the Royal Society's esteem.
His colleagues were searching for something
more meaningful. So he put the random
selection aside and suffered the migraine.

He went to his study and dissected
the smallest barnacles in the world, mere
specks of creatures. In one, strangely, the male
was a miniscule parasite that stuck
its whole life on the flesh of the female.
There must be a mistake. What kind of a God
would have chosen to create a species
like that? In which the male was nothing but
a degenerate, larva-like sac
with a sex organ! Darwin asked himself,
had the time come, finally, to explain
the simple truth? The ill-formed little monster —
to which he gave the name *Ibla cumingii* —
was every bit as perfect as man.

Icon of the Heavenly Ladder

Monastery of St. Catherine,
Sinai, 12th Century

The heavenly ladder climbs from the lower-left hand corner
to the upper right, where the Lord beckons from the gate
of heaven, which in this icon is a curved opening
in the golden horizon. This blessed figure
welcomes the pure of heart as they ascend the ladder,
their eyes lifted in rapture. The saints climb precariously,
threatened at every step by miserable dark angels,
harassing them with prods, lassos. When the pure weaken,
tempters terrorize their bellies.

Of the 26 figures, thus far only 7 have fallen
to their perdition, not such a bad proportion
for the Byzantine Empire. In the upper left-hand corner
a choir of magnificent angels observes the chain
and weakened links. Yea-sayers, even in their perfection,
are fraught with uneasiness concerning the fate of humans.
Inside a mountain stand the damned, huddled together,
encased like amber. They, too, wear sober robes and beards.
They, too, reach out their hands. One of the sinners
raises his hand so high that his fingers reach the rim
of damnation — but there is no sign of solace coming.

To the Mummy of a Thief in the Crypt of St. Michan's Church, Dublin

After six hundred years, the watery parts
are gone — intestines, muscle, liver, spleen.
Your lizard-like surface has turned turf brown.
Yet the wages of your sin remain —
stumped bones instead of hands, your single foot.
A thief, hung at last for your fourth offense.
We don't know why he's here, the sexton says,
interred in our church with saints. In the slot
above you, a knight, whose pickled body
was carried from the East. His crossed arms
embrace the absence of a sword. His last
Crusade. And lying stiffly in the dust
beside you is a 14th century nun.
She whom Christ once warmed with grace
lies snug now with not an inch to spare
against your sacrilegious arm. Your tale
is told in severed bones, but hers is gone.
Her cloister's stone is cobbled in the streets
of Dublin. *Some say it's chemicals that makes*
these bodies mummify, something in the ground
like gas. The sexton shakes his head. *Some say,*
it's grace. St. Michan's gift. A kind of miracle.
Who knows? He points us toward the steps.
Your head is propped between two bricks — its eyes
are talking to the nun. Does she believe
the tale you tell — I begged for bread; I stole to live?
Judge for yourself, the sexton says and slams
and bolts the heavy door. *I think it's gas.*

Keeping Dry

This drink costs ten bucks
behind brown drapes, where
I wait a rainy evening out,
reading
the illuminated text
of 53rd Street —

A man on the margin
steadies his cardboard box
by the niche
of a stone porch, and wraps
in his coats like a saint
in a winding cloth and slides
into his sepulcher
feet-first and pulls
a sodden plastic sheet
to plug the end. *It's a flood
out there, in all this rain,*
reports my friend,
jiggling her golden wrists
at fate. *How sad
that man is* — she misreads
my look — *But homeless choose
their own sad ends.*
Imagine that.
Imagine
my hero's cardboard coffin
floating from his own
flooded graveyard
into the ocean.
Imagine him *choosing*
(next time) to pilot a trim sloop's
rudder, sailing the horizon
happily ever after.

These Shards Are Wrist Bones

> In a religious dispute 300 years ago,
> Hopis from Oraibi destroyed the Christian
> village of Awatovi.

When I found these shards
scattered where rain embedded them,
wrist bones bound by baked dirt, roots, thistle,
cooking pots, corn meal pots, cracked,
smashed on rocks, and tossed
in a garbage heap beneath the village,

they were still connected
to cords of red peppers
that hung like claws above each doorway,
still connected to the night that Bear Clan,
Snake Clan, crouched in kivas,
the night men with cedar bark torches
came moaning *wah ou, wah ou*
and ran through the village,
tossing their bundles of lit sticks.

I return to Antelope Mesa
bearing these burnt pots, these angry bones,
these shards cleared of baked dirt
and kept for years in a box beneath my bed,
their red lines worn, their wavy anger worn.

Today I drive a jeep on frozen mud,
looking for a trace of Awatovi,
for a track that doesn't end at a rusty windmill
or at an abandoned hoghan
with a patch of snow on its sheltered side.

I come seeking peace, my brothers,
no longer the young man in jeans
with two kids and a topographic map,
no longer the young man looking for another way
to experience sadness or anger.

Returning to the same rocks near the flank
of your abandoned mesa,
I dig where moaning sounds — *Take them* —
and put them into the ground — *Take these shards* —
and cover them. *These are your wrist bones,*
and mine.

Don't Be Afraid, Gringo

It is no accident that your train
stalled in this switchyard,
nor that I cross the rocky arroyo
with a sling of firewood,
nor that I run toward your stalled train,
nor that I toss
this pebble to wake you.

Though the window is streaked and pocked
with dried desert rain, and smudged with hair,
it makes no difference. I see you.

I dance on a rail outside your window.
My shift balloons in the wind,
my arms beat like an agitated eagle.
I swing my thin butt the way the wealthy walk
the Reforma. This is no accident.

That I dance the dance you remember,
lanterns alight in the plaza,
mariachis crooning, that I am a child
and make faces as I dance,
gringo, this is not a random occurrence.

This is my home — the switchyard,
the siding beside the arroyo —
and you have come a long way to join me.
Let me put down my sticks.

As the train shudders, let me climb
the side of your Pullman
and press my face to your window.
I am Delores Rodriquez,
Torreon, Chihuahua, and I have chosen
this vulnerable time and lonely place.

Gringo, there is nowhere to go,
no one to turn to,
no one to dance with, but me.

Guam

It's gotten so you talk about Guam
every day now, but only the letters
and loneliness. For years
I've tried to pin particulars
to your life in the war — men you lived with,
comic incidents that must have made
the barracks livable, a texture to your
boredom. Once, you talked about the mud
that made Guam stick, but never spun a yarn
about the rain. The natives? They were
dirty thieves, but now they've stripped you
to the brain. You trembled with surprise
when I asked about the town. Searching
the mud behind your rheumy eyes for *town*,
you discovered none. The only story
you remember is your teeth and the pain
of their departure. The dentist stood his ground,
though. He kept you toothless in Hawaii
two months, until the dentures sent you
to Guam. The other tales have disappeared —
if ever formed — and Guam's become
a voiceless state of being for you, like hell
or heaven is, where you've returned at last
and left me by myself. I waited too long
to redeem the war we carried on,
father and son, for fifty years. Well,
closeness, touching, matter now, not anger.
I'll make up your stories later.

from

Medicine Stone

(2002)

Lachrymae Rerum

Fried flounder on cardboard plates, slaw,
drafts of dark beer. Pain has followed us here
to the fish place in Riverhead. I'm fed up
with clammers' shot backs, bad kidneys,
and their wives' arthritis. I'm fed up
with cancer wearing suspenders and dousing
its flagrant heart in wine. The tables here
are crammed with pain. The coolers
are stacked with eel like black,
pickled sausage. Go ahead, though, keep talking
about your cancer's source — the church
you grew up in, its Baroque Italian priest
and pinched nuns that scuttled across your youth
like bugs. You're not buying it, not an ounce
of original sin, not a word of Augustine,
nor anything that carries you down
from joy. That's what you *say*. Even the walls
of this joint are sweating blood, but you've
converted to a new belief — the cosmic dance.
Go ahead, keep talking. I'm not thinking now
about the sweating bodies of the dead
in Africa, nor that woman with the bomb
beneath her t-shirt in Sri Lanka, nor the kid
gunned down in Brooklyn, nor the arrogance
of righteous violence. I'm trying to imagine
the original blessing. Go ahead, tell me
the wizened eel of history is somebody's fault —
Jesus' or the popes' — and if left to ourselves
we'd surely dance. And be compassionate
and tender. Go ahead, finish your beer.
Let's kick up our heels. It's Saturday night
in any case, and I'm tired, too, of tears.

Sirens

What song the Syrens sang...
[is] not beyond all conjecture.
                    Sir Thomas Browne (1605-1682)

Their song is a generous wind
from the island's throat. Listen,
my friend. You must learn to forget
the violence you're accustomed to
and years of hapless voyage.

At first you can't imagine
a respite from discipline,
from the petulant telephone
telling its worst — of intractable
pain, unthinkable dread.

A respite from Alfred,
who never met the therapist
you sent him to, not once.
From all the petty coughs
and silent screams.

From Richard's desperate chest —
He has lost his job, his energy,
his hope. He doesn't know
where misfortune comes from,
but knows you'll make it go.

Your heart has claims of its own,
the Syrens sing. Abandon
discipline. Your body can't take
the knots it's tied in. Come closer,
we'll loosen them.

I'm Gonna Slap Those Doctors

Because the rosy condition
makes my nose bumpy and big,
and I give them the crap they deserve,
they write me off as a boozer
and snow me with drugs. Like I'm gonna
go wild and green bugs are gonna
crawl on me and I'm gonna tear out
their goddamn precious IV.
I haven't had a drink in a year
but those slick bastards cross their arms
and talk about sodium. They come
with their noses crunched up like my room
is purgatory and they're the
goddamn angels doing a bit
of social work. Listen, I might not
have much of a body left,
but I've got good arms — the polio
left me that — and the skin on my hands
is about an inch thick. And when I used
to drink I could hit with the best
in Braddock. Listen, one more shot
of the crap that makes my tongue stop
and they'll have something on their hands
they didn't know existed. They'll have time
on their hands. They'll be spinning around
drunk as skunks, heads screwed on backwards,
and then Doctor Big Nose is gonna smell
their breaths, wrinkle his forehead, and spin
down the hall in his wheelchair
on the way to the goddamn heavenly choir.

The Six Hundred Pound Man

Of the six hundred pound man on two beds,
nothing remains,
not the bleariness with which he moved his eyes
nor the warm oil curling in his beard.

Though the sheets and plastic bags are gone,
his grunts, his kind acceptance gone,
I see him now, rising in the distance,
an island, mountainous
and hooded with impenetrable vine.

When I awaken to the death
of the six hundred pound man
and cannot sleep again,
I paddle to his shore

in search of those flamboyant trees
that flame his flanks,
in search of bougainvillea
blossoming on his thighs,
of women who rise to touch him
tenderly with ointment,

in search of healers, singers
who wrestle souls of old bodies
back to bones, back to dirt, and back back
to their beginnings.

As I enter for the first time
this medicine circle,
bearing chickens in honor of the god,
words dancing from my lips,

spirit like the plume of a child's volcano
rises

and then the medicine, the medicine is good
and the tongues, the tongues are dancing
and the fathers, oh! the fathers are dancing

and this worthless and alien body,
this six hundred pound man,
I discover him beautiful.

The Man with Stars Inside Him

Deep in this old man's chest,
a shadow of pneumonia grows.
I watch Antonio shake
with a cough that traveled here
from the beginning of life.
As he pulls my hand to his lips
and kisses my hand,
Antonio tells me
for a man whose death
is gnawing at his spine,
pneumonia is a welcome friend,
a friend who reaches
deep between his ribs without a sound
and puff! a cloud begins to squeeze
so delicately
the great white image of his heart.

The shadow on his X-ray grows
each time Antonio moves,
each time a nurse
soothes lotion on his back
or puts a fleece between his limbs.
Each time he takes a sip of ice
and his moist chest shakes with cough,
the shadow grows.

In that delicate shadow
is a cloud of gas
at the galaxy's center,
a cloud of cold stunned nuclei
beginning to spin,
spinning and shooting
a hundred thousand embryos of stars.
I listen to Antonio's chest
where stars crackle from the past,
and hear the boom
of blue giants, newly caught,
and the snap of white dwarfs

coughing, spinning.
The second time
Antonio kisses my hand
I feel his dusky lips
reach out from everywhere in space.
I look at the place
his body was,
and see inside, the stars.

Brain Fever

reminds me of Sarah Gorecki
propped-up in bed, fluffed pillows
along her sides and her husband
in his chair by the black window
doing the day's crossword. She took
to bed the week they shut the mill
in Donora, which is exactly
how George remembers it —

coming home with his last check
already bit by a few drinks,
he found her under the comforter
whispering how cold she was.
What fits she had! One spell led
to another — red pills, the big
green pills, the gallbladder. At last
the neighbors stopped pestering her
and telling her she's getting stronger.

Sarah told me the brain fever
set in that summer like coffin fog
on a damp day by the river. It spread
deep behind her eyes and made her weaker
than a pigeon. George was a real
lifesaver, though. After thirty years
of staying out and cutting-up,
that man sure came down in a hurry.

The Pounds of Flesh

You weighed one hundred five the day
you married. It's been a battle since —
buttocks, abs — but you held fast until this.

You swat the child's hands from your hoops
and gold chain. Drooling, he makes you
wipe your blouse and failed thighs with juice

and your weightlessness hoists the burden
of gravity. *The pounds will disappear
in time,* I explain. If only she had faith

in natural law, Aquinas could show,
within a pound or two, her weight just fits,
but he's not here. I face her mass alone.

I want to say, Your orange scent is attractive,
as are your large breasts, no matter what size
your husband desires. Appearances are

deceiving, even when you can't see them.
I'm sure the weight will suddenly fade,
like much we prize in life, but I can't say when.

Death House

Each day your cluttered bed
reveals a different version
of the house you're making
of cardboard, balsa wood,
and the Popsicle sticks
your sister brought, a design
you sketched, but abandoned,
a dozen years back
because your wife had split
by then, and you were broke.

The house is crisp, every bit
as fine as those you built
for the rich in Southampton,
those eccentric retreats
erected for delight.
It's even better, you explain,
brushing a few slivers
of gluey debris
from your distended abdomen's
shelf, and showing me
the latest improvement
on your old design.

Today's touch
is a railing for the porch.
Yesterday's — a larger deck.
Last week you made a ramp
from the children's bedroom
to the pool. But tonight
you'll tear that feature out,
or add a window, or re-size
the molding.

When I come
again tomorrow morning
to talk about dying,
the house, like Penelope's shroud,
will be no closer
to completion, and you'll look
at the pile of cardboard and glue
on your table and tell me
you need more time. It's such a job
getting everything to fit
and you have to be patient.

Work Rounds: On Lines by Tomas Transtromer

The lessons of official life
go rumbling on.
We send inspired notes
to one another.

The parade of distracted figures slows,
eddies, and each slides an "s"
around the obstruction — a lorry
of breakfasts, a medicine cart.

I am looking at you, at the fringe of hair
you didn't pull tight. A shaft of sun
pierces the mountainous clouds in your eyes.
You must be bursting with news.

Has the man in the next room returned at last
from his journeying fever? Has he sent us
a message? You look to the chart
and show me, *Here is the culture. Negative.*

All these years I, too, have hoped for the same thing,
an inspired note. I am grateful for the gift
of your news. How unlikely
the improvement was! And for the messenger's grace.

Medicine Stone

This stone I picked at a medicine dance
on a cold June day near Wounded Knee.

In my bare feet, I carried this stone
into the circle of those with need.

A sun dancer danced in front of me,
touched my shoulder with a sprig of sage.

A sun dancer chanted in front of me
and blessed me with his medicine pipe.

Here in the city, the sky is brilliant.
I carry this stone in a buckskin pouch.

Here in the city, we suffer in private.
Each of us stands at the circle alone.

This stone is an aspect of soul that lasts.
This stone is a remnant of no account.

Here in the hospital, coyote is dead.
This small stone is of no account.

Wolves, spiders, moles, snakes, ants are dead.
This spherical stone is of no account.

Eagles, hummingbirds, ravens, bats are dead.
This stone is a remnant of no account.

Only the voices of suffering live,
the skin, and what happens beneath the skin.

Still, I carry this buckskin pouch
and a small stone wrapped in a wad of sage.

This stone is an aspect of soul that lasts.
I call it my friend, my black stone friend.

My Machine

If I had a machine to use
in a case like yours, I'd use it
on the nucleus that makes
my feelings, to deepen them.

I'd take a long time, like a monk
at morning prayer, before I spoke
and turn each word into a sign
of passion. When I told you,

yes, the damage is more
than anyone knew, I'd hold you
in my arms, desperately close
like death. I'd throw off the sham

of working in a reasoned way
to find the answers to your pain.
Instead, I'd use an archaic
neural poem and feel the pull

of healing, skin to skin, instead of
acting neither man nor woman
and doing the decent thing. The ache
would be a price worth paying.

The Shoe

Public Health Inspector
William Townsend, died 1968,
Black River, Jamaica

Townsend took a curve too fast
and died near the coast. Nobody heard
for hours. Every few minutes
I turned to the window and cursed him.
He won't come, I thought, *the bastard won't.*

The road from Maggotty came up
through curves of banana trees battered by rain,
but the sick arrived anyway.
Glistening loudly, they filled the clinic.
We walked up and down to quiet their babies.

I was witless with anger.
Townsend had promised to come at noon
and take us away — we had such
important work to do. *Americans!*
Sister clicked her teeth at my arrogance.

At Townsend's funeral, his father
held up a shoe and cried, *He walked
in the pathways of righteousness.* I sat,
rod straight, on a folding chair
at the front of the church and didn't speak.

For isn't righteousness the brother
I never had? In Babylon,
years later, I listen for the sound
of Townsend's step. For him to greet me
in clinic. I'll follow him anywhere.

Reverence for Life

At break time I sat on the loading dock
behind the rolling mill at Wheeling Steel
with a book about Albert Schweitzer
while my friends played poker.
A series of photographs showed him
on the porch of a ramshackle building;
at the bench of his famous organ
which, the caption assured, was lined with lead
to save his music from mildew.
A shot of a muddy river
with him on the landing; and a peculiar
photograph of the helmeted doctor
examining a child's leg, while a starched,
immaculate woman stood next to him,
a buoy of duty. Unaware
of how not to pose, she looked at the camera
for validation, as if to say, *Here I am
at the end of the earth, yet even so...*
but Schweitzer paid no attention.
His eyes were stuck on that festering leg,
labeled *elephantiasis*, but in those days
what good would a stare do, even his?
And so I imagined the gaze moving back
to the unnamed woman, *a European nurse,*
and her astonishment. When my break ran out,
Riel, the foreman, cuffed me across the hat.
Goddamn books, he growled. *Ain't worth shit.*

Accidental

for Nancy Taylor

George Eliot wrote, "It's never too late
to be who you might have been," a thought
that simmers like a sheen behind my eye
when you tell your story — For an hour
before he fell to his death, the boy
and his roommates gambled at a game
of spitting farther and still farther
from the second-floor balcony. He leaned
the last inch that he wouldn't have tried
if just then the beer hadn't hit him, or if
he had been a larger man, or less afraid
of seeming queer to his friends, or more
confident of passing his course in
Victorian Novelists. So he hawked
his glob more than a foot past the last mark
the others had made. At which point
the baseball cap that covered his pale, thin head
jerked into an arc above the railing,
and before there was time for the girls
who watched from the sidewalk to scream
or jump back, the top of his overturned skull
smashed into the edge of the concrete,
and the rest of his body flipped backwards
into the daffodils. This week, you say,
the students are looking into themselves
and carrying more weight than the chaplain
would like. Stunned by the exquisite campus,
I ask the names of flowering trees
around the lake. *This one*, you say, *is Judas*,
and the other — just as beautiful — I miss.

Scorpion

Arriving at sunset soaked from the road
and reeking of human chemicals,
the children neither awake nor asleep
and the heat unbearable, we took
what the bored senora said was the last
untaken room in town. On the tile
of the dripping shower, my daughter found
a humungous scorpion. *Squash it!* she cried,
an act I tried to avoid, as I knew
its slight resistance to death, the scrunch
of its carapace against my sole
would awaken a pain I hoped to forget
and so I took the children aside and said,
Scorpions are good. They eat the vermin.
Even the vermin are entitled to live
until eaten. The children found my opinion
amusing. *Come on, old daddyo,*
kill it, kill it. And then my 3-year-old son
charged in with a carved baseball bat, yelling,
Take that, Geronimo! Take that! Take that!
Without a further attempt to explain
life's interconnectedness, I stepped
on that alien thing, and with a ring
of enthusiastic witnesses
cheering me at the toilet, I flushed it.

Sir William Osler Remembers
His Call on Walt Whitman

I took the ferry that day and found him
in the front room of a small house
on Mickle Street, buried to his chest
in papers, magazines, and musty
brown bundles. *Push yourself a path,*
he said. *I reckon you're a friend of Bucke's.*

His famous head had aged majestically —
unkempt white beard; smooth, clear cheeks;
a fissured, geographic forehead.
His voice was pitched a shade too high,
but strong like the rest of him. Of symptoms
he said but little — remarkable

for a man of 65. For a moment
I felt that *sweet aromatic presence*
his disciples speak of — but for me, though,
it was the edge of chaos. I often wish
the man had made more of a difference
in my life, but how could I forego

restraint? Or become attached to a poet's
strong magnetic force? For a professional
like myself, his unruliness galled
and festered, though in the end I succumbed
to his charm and savored the music
of his tongue — but with restraint. I would not cross

the line between us, nor pass the gate that says,
Who enters here, abandons discipline.

Sunsets

I take him to the beach at sunset.
It's a production, pulling his body
from the front seat, half-carrying
his legs across the rocks, finding
a flat place to set his chair. Too late.
By the time we are set, sun is gone
and the last few layers of sky
are about to burn out.
                    When I was young,
I dreamed of taking him on trips,
the two of us. He wore pressed pants.
Me, a pigtail and safari hat.
We crossed a wilderness where lakes
breathe steam. We pitched our tent
in a hollow of needles
and talked about the war. *What is it, son,*
just between the two of us, you want
in life? He punched his jacket up,
stuck it behind his neck
and smiled.
                When I was young, I dreamed
we arrived at the beach with never a word
about the ugliness of circumstance
and with plenty of time before sunset.
The sky was glorious, and he could stand.

Chrysler for Sale

From the lucky postwar Nash
to the Olds he wrecked
the year before my mother died,
every car my father bought
was blue for the Blessed Virgin.

After the wreck, my mother
was never the same. She wouldn't set foot
in the Olds again, said it made
a funny noise. Just looking at it
brought back that night, brought back
that colored man with no insurance,
big, drunk and rude to the point of insolence.

So my father bought a steel gray Chrysler,
turbo engine, racing wheels
and vinyl top. He told her,
Don't be afraid. This car is a gift,
a miracle, just wait and see.

Propped tightly in her right front seat,
clutching her rosary beads,
my mother faced a maze of malls, ramps,
bridges, freeways and lengthy strips
until at last

the neighborhood changed
and the old apartments appeared, the sparkling
friends of long ago, friends before the war.
Look at this Chrysler! she called out.
Look at my Lee!
Look where he's taking me!

And they put down their highballs
and raised their eyes from the cards
as my father drove in his sleek steel Chrysler
through the old blue neighborhoods,
sitting erect, putting his hand on her knee
and telling her, It's all right, Peg. It's all right.

from

Bursting with Danger and Music

(2012)

Bursting with Danger and Music

With my window cracked a little,
the sealant allows a reed of sound
to penetrate the van —

kee-oo — as the road slashes
cuts in Pennsylvania's hills
of lacquered snow — *kee-oo* —

Tones from another world
unfreeze the tiny valves
of fossil crustaceans.

Uncover them! Drape the slopes
with iced instruments —
recorders, mouth harps, oboes, flutes!

Kee-oo, kee-oo, kee-oo, kee-oo,
reed of cicada,
wheedling of the humpbacked flute player.

His hump is bursting with seeds
he recklessly scatters
and grinds to a paste of cinders.

He splotches snow with showers
of black notes, he raises
an orchard from wilderness.

Peaches! Culture! Pumpkins! Beans!
Mounds of tough maize!
Powamu! Mudhead! Tewa! Corn!

In this February snow
I'm bursting with danger and music
I cannot control, O my soul.

Sewage Treatment

Visiting the sewage treatment plant
beside the Monongahela River
in Pittsburgh — that trip was surely
another of the million small betrayals
I suffered at the hands of teachers
who didn't understand anything
about medicine. I chalked it up
to their obsession with demanding
irrelevance. *Those who can't do, teach.*
And then they put sewage on the exam!

At the time I planned to become
a psychiatrist and later that summer
married my sweetheart, a definite plunge
into maturity. That lush grass,
that continuous thrum of machines
and clatter of catwalks. A uniformed flunky
took us to each step of purification,
from sludged to seraphic. Today,
I'm imagining those pipes and pools
continually refreshed by filtering,
aeration and slime, enabling
the past to flow into me, more wholesome
and drinkable than when it happened.

Grease

What he remembers about those pits
below the rolling mills at Wheeling Steel
is loads of spent grease that had no way out
unless lifted through a hatch at the top
by bucket. The hatch was big enough
for one to crawl through — cloying stench
of muck to the calves of his boots, oilskin
glistening with molten rivulets,
a bucket's suck as it cleaves the grease's
surface. He clamped each half-filled bucket
to the cable and tugged for his up-side
companion to haul it up. The first few
were easy, but then that queasiness
rose in his caw, and he began to collapse
under the coils of steel rolling thinner
and thinner above his head. He buckled
under their whipping in loud silver bands,
their oily sheen, their brutal power, the ingots,
volcanic rivers. In that nausea
of grease he struggled to make himself
smaller, zero, nothing, but the sweetly
viscous substance was too much. Wavering,
green, his eyes about to vomit, he climbed
from the pit before his hour was up
and sat on the bench for the rest of the day,
head down, elbows on his knees. Some of the men
slapped him on the back. They told him stories
and one of them brought him soup.

Deep Structures

I never knew how deep the structures were
or why the names for them intrigued me so.
Amygdaloid — the sound tripped off my tongue.
And *hippocampal gyrus* made me sing.

The music of these names intrigues me so,
though the tendons of my hand — forgotten all.
And *hippocampal gyrus* makes me sing,
for thirty years still dancing from my tongue.

The tendons of my hand — forgotten all,
as are the layered structures of my back.
Yet thirty years of tumbling off my tongue —
those rhythmic nebulae within my brain.

The muscled structures of my back are zip.
But *caudate, red,* and *pallidum* survive —
those rhythmic nebulae that strum my brain.
Gone, passion that I had for listing names.

But *caudate, red,* and *pallidus* endure,
and *amygdaloid*, an almost perfect self.
Gone, passion for obsessive naming names,
but those archaic structures still grip firm.

Amygdaloid is almost perfect self.
And even though I judged my soul was lost,
those deep archaic structures never budged,
but form the links by which our lives connect.

And even though I judged my soul was lost
I never knew how deep its structures were,
their buried links by which our lives connect.
Amygdaloid! It dances from my tongue.

from *The Internship Sonnets*

1.

Orientation. He appeared at seven,
welcomed by a voice, *You don't belong,*
a repetitive warning that no one
heard but him. The Chief arose. A strong
odor of eagerness arrived. The other
interns smiled and shrugged; their faces eased
by conversation, a band of brothers
being forged. He looked down, took a piece
of paper and scribbled, *I'm terrified*
to start. How about you? But put it between
some pages. Whom to trust? Could he rely
on their eye contact? His neighbors' keen
gazes slid by. Not one of them saw him.
He chose to keep his feelings hidden.

2.

Nearly every word they said became real,
although much of it remained internal —
a cutting jibe that caused a nurse to feel
angry and hollow, or a soft fraternal
phrase, so precious because unexpected.
The only faith they had was flesh-and-bones,
organic they called it, and they rejected
patients' sufferings and stories as
functional, so that when they diagnosed
they had no idea their words became
characters in patients' worlds and pierced
their hearts and grew spines. They were children
playing doctor with puzzles and machines.
Eager for their ends, they lacked the means.

3.

The rule on the ward team was pledging
fealty to the chief. Violations,
like telling patients the truth, or hedging
on unnecessary tests, or vacations
from the floor, were dealt with severely.
The chief said, *Honey, the surgeons got it all.*
A piece of cake. Or, *Stan, you nearly*
died, but everything's fine. It was small,
nothing to worry about. Then discreetly
withdrew. After which, patients burst
out with, *What?* Or a timid *"why?"* tucked neatly,
sotto voce. To whom was the intern's first
duty? Continents of pain. Callow youth.
Hippocrates said nothing about truth.

5.

Cold spaghetti and thirty-two ounces
of Coke at midnight supper. A littered
foursome, in which the quietest announced
he had another hit. The embittered
second stabbed his plastic tray with his pen.
The third intern shuffled through a stack
of index cards; his wife's father in Johnstown
had just died of cancer. The last attacked
a stale Portuguese roll with his fork.
Gears grinding, motors turning, but nothing
happening. The ozone-like smell of stale work.
Did they suffer from sleep deprivation?
Thirty-six on and twelve off, a sublime
method of learning the value of time.

8.

The patient is a thirty-six-year-old man
in his usual state of good health
until yesterday morning when he began
to have ureteral pain. Nothing helped,
not even his mother-in-law's codeine.
Excruciating. The ER sent him home
with a chit for the clinic, after finding
a stone in his urine. Later, they combed
his old chart and found a film from last year
that showed a lung nodule. No one had called
him in. Now the mass has gotten bigger
and he's lost weight. It looks like we've killed
our chance for a cure. We admitted him
for a work-up. The prognosis is grim.

9.

The indigents were placed in open wards,
thirty-two beds, beneath a maze of rods
and drapes that slid across, unless ignored,
to create private space, or the façade
of privacy. First floor, men; women above.
Heads near the wall and feet adjacent
to the aisle. A umbrous gallery of
portraits hung above the beds. The complaisant
noblesse oblige of it all. During rounds,
the chief in charge, the doctors said *ma'am*
and *sir*, while scavenging beneath brown
skin for carrion. An objective exam,
nothing personal. *The patient is a poor
historian*, they groaned. This lacks a cure.

11.

Interned: To be coerced into a camp
and made to work, because of who you are.
To be Japanese-American during the war
and considered a traitor. To be clamped
into preventive detention, as Boer
women and children were by British
soldiers. Incarcerated. Diminished.
An alien about to be sent. The score
was hospital, eleven months; interns,
zero. He thanked the Good Lord for gifts
of resilience, appetite, and the swift
embrace of sleep. After which, he returned
to the world with a jolt — knocked out of bed
by a buzzer. Inclement weather ahead.

12.

Five-forty-five, the twenty-sixth of June,
and Elizabeth Bishop is on his desk.
At last the rumbling of the storm is gone.
Early twilight. Seven of the last
eight days it stormed, almost a record,
but not quite. He was feeling that surge
of grace a good day gives. In his restored
future, he could see his genius emerge,
his fortune soar beyond his rented rooms,
infested stairwell, and broken chandelier.
Elizabeth Bishop, in one of her poems,
has the prodigal son, at the end of his year
in a pig sty, returning. Look at me come,
after a long absence, I'm arriving home.

That Intern Dream

I had that intern dream again last night,
white coat and pants, but I'm decades older
than the group of docs I hadn't met.

In the middle of the scene, I kept
clutching a fear so tight, my smile was tin,
but I hadn't seen a single patient yet.

At midnight the rumpled interns ate
cold spaghetti, bread and juice. In a seat
across the room, I scanned their faces,

convinced they hadn't seen my grievous sin
of never having learned to put
a tube in place or make an incision.

Instead I read my books. Emergency!
My name was called. A code. I had to run,
but didn't know in which direction.

The route I took was wrong, and I reversed.
My coat and shirt went down. My pants collapsed.
I skimmed along in underpants and socks.

The call was cardiac. If there had been
a chance of saving face, it went. The patient
gasped for breath, but I had never seen

a cath put in or learned resuscitation.
Crowded around his bed stood eyes
that relished the confusion. Nothing

worked. And then the dream resolved
in gratitude: my own body, my own bed,
my secret still secure, nobody dead.

Virginia Ham

December isn't the same
since Mary Johnson's ham
packed in Styrofoam and ice

with packets of pancake mix
and slabs of frozen bacon
has stopped arriving.

A furnace in Mary's chest
had burned so fiercely hot, I swore
she wouldn't last that year,

let alone the next. And next.
By chance or prayer, but not
by me, the passion

of her white cells lessened,
the fire was quenched, and she
began to breathe again.

It wasn't long till Mary ran
from our slagheap northern town
to a condo on the coast.

For 13 years the ham,
steaming with dioxide ice,
appeared on my porch

around December first,
until instead its absence came
and said she'd gone.

All Souls' Day

So much depends on this frail old man
who lurches from his seat – *I'm next!* –
and works his cane across the room.

He purses his lips, like a clarinetist
leading a parade among the graves
on All Souls' Day. So much depends

on the white elastic rim of shorts
that shows above his belt, on the cap
he swoops above his speckled head,

Hey, doc! I'm almost there! Whether
I pick up my instrument and dance
behind him, or spread my picnic

on a white sarcophagus, or just
carry my dead inside, so much
depends on this frail old man

who swivels his bad foot forward,
loudly chewing, almost swallowing
the sharp black notes of his clarinet.

Darkness Is Gathering Me

On a line by Alphonse Daudet

False spring is making its rounds this morning.
Darkness is gathering me into its lair.
It's twilight and my nurses are speaking —
You'd think they were talking about flowers.

Darkness is gathering me into its lair
but it isn't unpleasant. I imagine
it's morning, and my nurses are speaking
in a warm meadow. I have no business

imagining, but it's not unpleasant,
the way the nurses say, *It's a lovely wound...*
In that meadow, a wound has no business
turning a sulfurous color and dying.

The way the nurses talk, the lovely wound
is my morning, my body, my daffodils
abloom in sulfurous colors. I'm dying
but loveliness isn't. Let them run laughing

into the morning. My bloody daffodils
and sweetly rotting smell, what a case
of loveliness! I'll scamper, laugh
and hoot and dance in their wake.

Those sweetly-smelling nurses! My rotten case
is nailed shut. When the morphine wears off,
where will hooting and dancing be? At my wake?
Their bodies are firm; I wish I could touch them.

When the morphine wears off, they'll nail me shut.
False spring is making its rounds this morning.
Their bodies are firm; I wish I could touch them.
It's twilight and my nurses are speaking.

Detached Concern

My doctor's not engaged enough
to touch my hand. I wonder where
her feelings are, the human stuff.

My doctor doesn't take much guff
from wimps like me. Whatever care
she gages up, it's not enough.

Detached concern is less than tough.
It's thin and weak and pulseless, bare.
The human feelings screw its stuff.

The pains I feel are fairly rough.
Detached, my doctor wouldn't dare
engage them. They're not clear enough

to measure with her scope and cuff.
Her brow is knit, her white coat there,
but touching isn't — human stuff.

This illness wears me down. I slough
my hope in layers. Unaware,
my doctor's not engaged enough.
She hides her feelings, does her stuff.

Cosmic Sonnets

for Anne

1.

A spasm of loneliness grips my
esophagus — I wish it were otherwise.
On my side of the phone, the lousy
old forest sinks into darkness and silence.
On your side, the illuminated kitchen
blazes with liveliness, and in the hum
of your eager voice, I imagine
a slim piece of our separation
sawed off and the two ends brought nearer
together. I see us as Siamese twins,
joined at the chest, sharing one heart. I fear we're
predictable, dated, and too damn
intense, which leads me to contemplate
just how our beginnings made us that.

2.

What does a Big Bang mean? A speck
an astronomer picked up has spent thirteen
billion years in transit. They accept
it as a type of relic from the time
the universe spun from a thin ocean
of monotony to the lumpiness
that created *things*. The scent of lotion
on your hands, the unintended caress
of your fingertips brushing my lower arm,
my gratitude at spinning in an orbit
that nurtures life, your well-worn alarm
when I ask questions like, Does any of it
mean anything? Or are we going anywhere?
I don't know, but please stay, until we're there.

3.

The bang couldn't have been *big*. Dimension
didn't exist until the event
had occurred; nor, for that matter, time.
In retrospect, after a moment
had elapsed, the bang had to be minimal,
a *ping*, since ten to the minus ten of space
was all there was. We struggle with scale
in love as well. We think: How ardent the chase!
How deep! How eternal! But I've noticed
our conversations are sparser than they were
and quieter. As you sit in the Lotus
position, across from my computer
desk, you're bathed in glorious photons, *ping*,
oblivious to the original Bang.

4.

In the beginning there was a one
dimensional loop, and now — all this.
After the Bang came time, division,
loss and pain, in turn. Once anonymous
stuff lined up to receive a name and voice.
Philosophers say that chaos is deaf
to suffering, to our lack of choice
in the world, the terrible odds. Every breath
we take is troubled. There's evidence
enough for despair, but instead we choose
to love. What a paradox! You wince
at physics and can't carry a tune, but who's
more of a lovely song? When I forget
the music of the spheres, you bring it back.

5.

In the first ten to the minus eleven
of the universe's story, the plot
was complete, its dramatic tension
a sham. But the fact is, we have not
deciphered the text. In the Theory
of Everything, we've lost at least seven
dimensions along the way — fairy
universes. Only the brushfire of time
and the trinity that makes up space
remain — quasars, stars, and planets where
we live, but your presence, my love, creates
a twelfth, yet first, dimension, a rare
unbroken symmetry — call it *Dance* —
which enlivens space and time and chance.

Midnight Romance

On the midnight train from Moscow to Petersburg
we aim for romance: a milky glass of tea
straight from the samovar, the boreal forest
sliding backward beside our compartment window,
a uniformed steward to serve shots of vodka
for us to knock down, our two pale bodies
tangled on crisp sheets. But we stumble
into an airless sleeper packed with partially dressed
Orthodox priests and their elbows and abdomens,
and an angry conductor twists us into
another car and drops us into berth
#6, like stunned turtles in a terrarium.
The French in #5 and the pair of Texans
whose #7 is dirtier than their horses' stalls
rub broken glass into their grief outside our door.
We just aim for relief, but giant mosquitoes
prick us, especially you, and the toilet's odor
is heavier than virtue, and our attendant
smokes behind a newspaper in his seat. Shall I ask
about the comfortable climate control
in the brochure? Or mention the lack of towels
to the tank-like woman who barks at him?
And you promise me — with twelve volcanic bites
and your face already swollen —
you'll die of anaphylaxis before we arrive.
Why doesn't anything work? You insist that I
or the repellant, equally impotent,
smash something, anything. The embedded sweat
of thousands of Soviets seeps from every surface
and surges against our window. Wrapped
in woolen blankets right up to our faces, we eat
the last of the cheese and granola bars. The train
shudders and a voice announces in Russian,
Attention! Romance is about to begin.

Phrenology

Concavities and lumps above my ear
speak narratives I never would have known
before relentless loss of all my hair

turned truth about my scalp so baldly clear —
the story of my life is in the bone.
Convexities and slumps above my ear

identify the site of passion: here.
Like tenacity and hope, it's in a zone
invisible before the loss of hair

writ large the heady script of character.
Depression, fancy, awkwardness intone
complexity that's bunched above my ear

for you to read. Your gentle fingers, dear,
interpret my desire and mine alone.
My scalp is blessed to have no trace of hair.

It shines with gratitude — I love your care
for this old scalp, though never have I won
a way to read the bumps above *your* ear,
which even now are swathed in silver hair.

Astonishment

In memory of John Stone,
poet and physician

John, *enthusiasm* means possession
by the gods. To chisel the lines, to snap
your clauses into joint, to question
which word is most elegant and apt,
requires patience, detail, craft. But the juice
you pump into their hearts, the baritone
passion of your spleen, your antic voice —
these matter most. Your lungs grown
silent, astonishment still breathes in the lines
of your poems. You said the heart leads, the head
explains. Maybe, but its explanations
leave a lot to be desired. John, the spread
of grace is patchy at best, but your voice
enhances it. *Therefore, let us rejoice.*

He Lectures on Grace

The first setback to his talk
on grace was the lack
of sync between his laptop
and their projector.
An electronic screech
pierced the room, but when
at last they found a man
to fix the sound, it lessened
a little. And the glitch
in his introduction
by a ponderous former dean,
who mistakenly called him
a family doctor from
Missouri, while holding
the podium up with bursts
of hot gas, and then left
for his important meeting
before the talk — that could
have been worse. And the lunch,
a catered spread of salads,
sandwiches, schmoozing,
and lack of attention, didn't
actually prevent him
from speaking. Faces arose,
faces fell, the clatter
resumed. How he relished
this lesson in detachment!
And began, *Courage, said
Ernest Hemingway,
is grace under pressure.*

He Lectures at the Heritage Association Dinner

After dessert, the women
arranged themselves upstairs
in a private room. He began
by presenting the usual
distinction between letting
a patient die and killing.
His examples generated
a spark that ignited
tiny firecrackers behind
a dozen faces and waving
hands rose, *Doctor! Doctor!*
A husband suffering torture
long after his body
gave out — a physician's hubris.
An injured brother severed
from machines too soon
by doctors who had stolen
his wife's consent.
Passion took hold of the group.
Anger and urgency tore
great hunks of experience
from the women's hearts
and grief uncovered its roots.
Having sprung the hinges
of ethics, he sampled
the best dose in his cabinet —
silence. When passion subsided,
the president praised the talk
that had not been given
and thanked him profusely
for sharing his wisdom.

William Carlos Williams Circumcises
Ernest Hemingway's First Son

So I said, sure, and why not? The next sweet
       morning of Paris
              drunk with the warm scent
of rain on gravel
       in Luxembourg Gardens
             and my head as big as a bucket
a — shall we say — aftereffect
       of the prizefights we went to
             the night before
the four of us
       roiled in the grit and sawdust and sweat
             – Kill him!
             Kill the bastard! — Flossie cried.
So I picked up my leather kit and went back
       to Hem's flat
             laid the kid on the kitchen table
and lopped off his foreskin
       — *his teeny binky*, Hadley cried —
             which in those days
was what you did. At the sight of Bumby's blood,
       bloody big Hem
             standing at the side of the table
             holding the kid's head
 collapsed
       a sack of potatoes, a tin of lard
             fainted *ker-boom*
dead to the world. After the days in Paris
       they kept asking me
             how could I go back
to the pale complexities of practice?
       To the grime
             of Rutherford's bodies?
The drum of routine —
       I think of Hem on the floor at the first drop
             of his son's blood.
What a man! It isn't anything
       I could explain, I tell them. It's just
             making a living.

Delicate Procedures

for Jack S.

You scold me for pretending
doctors aren't as bad as they seem
and remind me I didn't appear
in Vietnam — my mantle
of privilege, complicity
of silence, cowardice, and the shell
I've built to protect myself.
We sit in our booth at the
Hi Lite Diner with mixed grill
and barbequed ribs. You have
your autopsy instruments.
I have my stethoscope and scalpel.
You begin with a standard
Y-incision — in a minute
my heart's on the table. I listen
for the scratch of shrapnel
in your posterior lung fields.
You tag my pump for later,
then sever my lungs from their
attachments and weigh them.
I make my initial cut
under the lip of your left
fifth rib, teasing the shards
of metal embedded there.
Experienced prosectors,
we complete our procedures
before the pie arrives. You reckon
you'll wait until we meet again
to get my brain. I hand you
some bloody shards from your back
on a napkin and collect
my organs. We split the bill.
In the parking lot we shake hands,
anxious to go home and begin
putting ourselves together again.

Do No Harm

Lights on. A spider in the sink is stunned.
Big sucker, hairy, brown. The body
bulges. Otherwise, it's squat. If I stand
a minute without moving, it'll glide
across the porcelain, attending
to its needs. Why do spiders appear?
This one lowered itself on a thread
that's gone. Exploring? It couldn't have been.
Spiders don't. Attracted to moisture?
The sink's dry now, but vulnerable
to flood. This arachnid is as good as dead.
What kind of being? I have no way
of understanding how it feels. It may eat
its own eggs. It hasn't friends. The sheen
of the porcelain means nothing to it.
Act without thought. I will turn the tap
to the left and pull out my razor.
Shouldn't I snap off the light and wait
for the spider to leave? Or flick it
gently with a Kleenex? I don't. I let
the torrent loose and turn to the shower,
so I can't see the spider struggling
and sliding on porcelain. For all I know
its whole life flashes in front of it.

Toenails

Plasters of fungus, horny planks
of keratin, replace toenails
that never meant a whit to me
until they thickened and went gray.

The podiatrist shrugs with indifference
at their display. *Consider the length
and burdens of treatment,* he muses.
It's true my toenails spend their days

encased in shoes, so why attempt
to salvage their integrity? My body
blossoms with dozens of losses,
each more convincing than the last,

so why waste enthusiasm
on pink, pliable nails, when I could
spend it for a younger, steadier heart,
a deeper, more distinguished face?

Pedal hope — a quest proportionate
to my place in the world, the way
of the Tao, awaiting some small life
to poke its chin from stony ground.

Theology

On our trip across the continent
I had intended to explain
all that I had learned about God,

but in the back seat the baby
couldn't stop screaming for relief,
so we fed and cuddled her

from Saskatoon to California.
When she finally threw in the towel,
I jumped to the top of my list,

the proofs of God's existence,
to which you listened less than a minute.
Whereof we cannot speak,

Wittgenstein wrote, *we must
remain silent.* Vermillion streaks
above the horizon,

Mount Shasta's darkened symmetry,
the fertile cloak of stillness
I hadn't yet put on. The road

frowned at me like a favorite aunt
whose grim face twitches
and collapses in laughter.

A Theory of Labor

for Elizabeth Rose

For the seventeenth hour
you heave and sweat,
as a soon-to-be son
butts your cervix, stretched
but stuck. Desperate
to push the Other out,
your pelvic floor
falters, its muscles
contract, even rip
if it comes to that. So this
is the price of our taste
of fruit from the tree
of knowledge of good
and evil, the taste that built
a vault-like skull and a brain
with a place for the future.
Yes, this is the price
of narrowing the loop of bone
you stand on — no birth
without pain. Collin
butts his head against desire,
a drum you share. It's old news
we're disproportionate.
Labor doesn't make sense,
not like the swift appearance
of apes, gorillas, chimps
into this Garden
of Paradise. Daughter,
you'd think by now
God would have given up
his pique about the taste
of forbidden fruit
and softened your bed
of roses, but as yet he hasn't.

Levitation

I follow Fifth four miles to the park,
cut to the brick road that skirts the zoo
and descends to the jam at the bridge
where I up the down ramp. If I'm lucky —
which is to say, not tied to rehearsing
the day's mistakes, or imagining myself
vindicated, or receiving a prize
for devoting my life to service —
I levitate, my soles fly from the sidewalk,
buoyed by firm air, as if balloons
without skins were rolling an inch or two,
sometimes three inches from fractured concrete.
Each time I pinch my thigh. *Snap out of it!*
But I don't. Never in life. My brain's a bird
not a dinosaur. I wave to the guards
at Aspinwall school and skip like a girl
on the path between First and Emerson.
How normal it feels to gravitate upwards,
to skim tops of the weeds, to shed my
dejection and awkwardness, and to ride
the maelstrom almost, but not quite, safely.

from

The Wound Dresser

(2016)

On Reading Walt Whitman's "The Wound Dresser"

You dampen dressings with warm water,
detach them from dried blood and debris,
carefully removing layers of gauze
without a gown, without gloves. An attendant
stands behind you with a bucket of soiled
bandages and shifts impatiently
from one foot to the other while you work.

You lean close to a soldier's yellow-blue
countenance, inserting his shattered language
into a letter addressed to his sweetheart.
When his whisper drops off, you suggest,
though never in haste, a word for the text.
You camp on a stool beside the cot,
observing your man, embracing the scene.

I stop at the foot of each cot and check
its numbers and charts. This body, wasted
and sinking, is next. I ask and record,
examine and plan, confident that signs
I interpret tell the truth. You remain
tinkering at your soldier's side, as I step
to the next cot and the cot after that.

The Secret of the Care

In those days I wore vestments to clinic —
pressed white pants, crisp shirt and jacket,
symbols of purity, though magnets
for stains, pockets puffed with instruments
and memory aids. I began by asking
questions, while fumbling my notes.
I squinted into the patients' lenses
for sclerotic vessels. I palpated
their abdomens, ballotted their livers,
and listened to respiratory crackles,
while disguising the depth of my doubt
with a kindly, but serious look.
It was difficult. I was surprised to find
how much I disliked some of the patients —
rude and demanding, manipulative,
violent and dense. Shrinking violets
that made me squirm. Paranoid addicts.
And a few that goaded my deep anger.
I tried to remember to step away.
The secret of the care of the patient,
professors had told me, *lies in caring*
for the patient, a maxim I was certain
cut to the core of healing. In time,
I convinced myself, all this rigmarole
of anger and hurt would work itself out.
I'd grow in wisdom. I'd ascend
to a higher, more open plane. Headache,
anger, fatigue, and doubt would disappear.
It's bound to get easier, I thought.

Take Off Your Clothes

I was taught to include specific
detail, like *down to your underpants
and socks*, or *all but your panties
and bra*, whichever might apply.

And season my request with modest
withdrawal, *I'll step out of the room
for a moment now.* And follow this
with the obvious, *Then I'll come back.*

I was taught always to offer a gown,
frequently folded backwards and faded,
and tell the patient, *Put the opening
behind. Put this sheet across your lap.*

In the next step, I learned to uncover
the roots of bewilderment, beginning
with the eyes and continuing down,
a performance laden with gesture,

encouraging hope. I delivered my script.
And you, my intimate companion,
you were consigned to endure the suspense
of me reading a narrative in your flesh.

Anita and Vladimir

Anita, whose course of radiation
hasn't sprung the tiniest leak
in her character, tells me the blues
that crawl each morning into her bed
are masculine. The icicle jitters
that slip under her skin by evening
are feminine. She gets rid of the men
by belting *What a Friend We Have
in Jesus* until the nurses come
and shush her. She relies on the Spirit
to hustle petulant women
out of the room. Anita's calm.

Vladimir, whose battle with cancerous
marrow has taught him to dissect
the brain's intoxicated tics,
wags a pear-shaped head made shiny
by steroids. I expect him to explain
Anita's deficits — superstition,
dullness, delirium. Last evening
in the family room, he lectured
on chemo to his roommate's daughter
until she turned away. I'm shaken
when Vladimir kisses Anita's hand.

The Silk Robe

... the white baubles and silk stockings of
your actresses excite my genitals.
Samuel Johnson, backstage at the Drury Theater

There's little excitement under the skin
of these bright halls. Though much of the flesh
is female, it's doughy from blockage
and muddled with wounds. The corridors'
odor — a confusion of solvents, seepage,
and hundreds of intimate chemicals.
Lit from behind by the bathroom light,
your blue silk robe has no place in this picture.
The scent you wear — Samsara, Gardenia,
Chanel? — is alien. When I walk in
your expression is amazed it's morning again
and I've returned to examine
your perfect chest. Perfect, except for
the swishing and rasping endocarditis.
I notice the flowered barrettes in your hair,
the creamy coolness you must have just
put on, your fingers asking me to sit.
Another two weeks, I explain, *of bed rest*
and intravenous. In here the drama
belongs to others, patients whose stories
twist into bitterness or blossom into gain
before going home. Nothing about you
fits the scene. Not the gauze clutching your groin
where they snaked a catheter up to your heart.
Not your toenails, painted maroon,
nor the delicate gold chain. There's not much
danger now — for you. Your cultures are clean.
You're upright and walking the halls.

Corrigan and the Giant

What victory! Corrigan's lymphoma
has melted away with an extract
of periwinkle like the Wicked Witch
in the *Wizard of Oz*. Corrigan's tumor
had bulged behind his breast and twisted
his trachea. He suffered night sweats
and matted nodes. What were the odds
his final scan would come out clear?

I dream about St. Christopher
carrying Corrigan on his shoulders
across the river. Far from the shore,
the compassionate giant pauses,
harried by venomous fish of doubt.
Will the saint continue his trek
toward heaven, or return Corrigan
to the world? Leaning against his staff,
Christopher resigns himself to returning
the man.
        When Corrigan meets me
the next morning, he's dashing to depart.

The Exterior Palace

Dressed for cocktails at noon, Mrs. Devlin
greets me by putting her whiskey down
while raising herself with her quad cane.
My entrance — her nurse's cue to complain
about her patient's tantrums and rejections.
I lean on a lovely couch in the sunroom,
listening to the nurse's soprano line —
still drinking despite strict instructions,
copping smokes, flouting compliance.
Below it, a contralto line — *Doctor,*
we need to get rid of this bitch of a nurse.
Tools of the trade fill my bag, but nothing
to set this brokenness right. The nurse,
I suppose, is driven by trust in the power
of words to enlighten and of reason
to sweep the deck. My patient flirts
and gossips and believes I'll wink
at her badness. She thinks I'm not
permitted to divulge our secret —
her internal palace, beyond its moat
and portcullis, beyond the magnificent
central court is a dank, unheated place.
Neither of us goes there. I'm enjoying
a delicate pattern of sunlight
across the rug and six framed photos
of different sizes that show her smiling.

Metamorphosis at Starbucks

Knobs appear beneath a drab sweater.
Then he comes in wearing a dark skirt
and gypsy blouse. When he sits at a table
near me, I notice the scarlet nails.
In a short time, I switch to the pronoun
she prefers. Several mornings a week
we sit, our backs to the windows,
two tables apart. When a story appears
in the *Times* on a marvel of medicine,
she brings it to my attention,
addressing me as "Doctor." I'm surprised
her voice hasn't softened. Her poise remains
masculine. Her breasts become larger,
but her face and arms, though smoother,
reveal the same sharp scaffolding.
With regard to an article
that touts advances in gene therapy,
she becomes flustered at my lack
of enthusiasm. With regard to a piece
about a theatrical new cure
for depression — I suggest reserving
just a pocket of doubt. In the months
that follow, her salt-and-pepper hair
remains dull, her makeup impasto,
her posture graceless. Metamorphosis
has ground to a halt, though trinkets of change
continue to accumulate. Each morning
I look for a difference I can't put my
finger on, but have faith will shine through
when it happens. I yearn to nudge her,
to tip her toward happiness. She's not
like those miracles in the paper; she's real.

Lift Up Your Heart

An ER treatment room at 2 AM.
On a gurney, a mangled body
cops brought in — *resisting.*

Awakened from a stupor, the beast
curses me, straining at straps
across his chest and hips. His vision

bleeding — confusion, fear, loathing.
Muscles at the back of my neck tense,
fingernails scrape across slate.

A package of tools on a tray.
As I begin to stitch the edges
of the man's wound, he twists his head,

spits at my too-close face, a glob
hits my eyebrow; a second, my mask.
No let-up. The cops will soon be back

to process my patient
and put him into the system
he resisted.

If I squeeze a portion of my heart
in a press, will a few drops
of compassion drip into my cup?

Ralph Angelo Attends the Barbeque

At the St. Charles Nursing Home barbeque picnic,
Ralph Angelo, wearing his signature straw hat,
strains his neck toward Gary, the man with a mike
and Hawaiian shirt, who badgers us to clap
to the thrumming boom box on a chair beside him,
chanting, *Heart of my heart   I love that melody.*
Ralph holds a tissue in each hand. He presses one
against the side of his veined nose, the other
to the crease of his mouth to collect his drool.
On Ralph's tray are plastic cups of thickened juice
and pureed hamburger. *Heart of my heart   brings back
a memory.* I feed him. Gary ribs the crowd
for not jumping to dance in the meadow, a joke
that falls flat. When Ralph puts his lips in motion,
they glide like snails across bricks. His puff
of consonants disappears below the drone.
His vowels die off. I kneel and put my ear
near his mouth to listen, but Ralph's lips
resemble a body being pulled toward the ground
while hanging from nails in the entryway.
Embarrassed, I ask Ralph what he means,
but his stony lips, his watery eyes,
fail to disclose, and Gary continues *Oh,
you beautiful girl   You great big beautiful girl.*
Volunteers passing by us distributing ice cream cups
remind me of the frozen chasm between us.

Skinwalkers

In these old buildings
deaths accumulate.
Though each is transparent,
it leaves behind a taste
of someone, a skinwalker.

In a bustling elevator
I'm surrounded by skinwalkers
who want to assist me.
They look antiseptic
and distracted, like people

doing and touching
the things they remember.
Some sip their coffee and smile.
Some steer their IV poles
like bishops' holy crosiers.

The skinwalkers mumble,
G'morning, when they jostle
and bump me, so closely
their touch is a lotion
that clings to my raw hands.

Hardly anyone remembers
the dead can't harm us.
Hardly anyone notices
these faint souls, flickering
with traces of sympathy.

Ockham's Razor

Ockham's razor shaves
stories to their cores,
its stainless blade relieves
complexity — and cures.

I want to say *zebra*,
the razor makes it *horse*.
I imagine a plethora,
am urged a single course.

Simplicity makes sense.
Discarding underbrush,
the secret of success —
a secret, too, of loss.

My rogue imagination
colors, enhances.
My ear yearns to listen,
my thalamus dances.

So — Ockham's razor sits
no longer trusted
in my medicine cabinet,
abandoned and rusted.

Poem for David

The day you died your sheepish letter came
begging me to write Dilaudid for the pain.
On flying home — your goddamn migraines
back again. After the second bleed
your mother was as good as dead, your dad
a wreck. You begged me to forgive your sick
activities last year, frightening my kids,
bringing meth into my home. *I'm clean,*
you wrote, *Rehabbed in the Vets for months.*

Your drowning made the local Evening News —
a body bobbing at the rocks a quarter mile
beyond the rapids. Swimming when a seizure
took him. An accident, they said. But no.
You hated water, had never learned to swim.
Heroin, Dilaudid, meth. Your manic flight
to help the victims of explosions, earthquakes,
fires — your merciless adrenalin.
Chaos and emptiness tracked you home.

In our Appalachian town, I stood like wax
beside your open casket. Above you —
an arrangement of roses from a woman
named Terri. I hovered near the guttered flame
your father had become, recalling the months
you spent tending the wounded in Vietnam,
your endless shifts in hospitals back home.
I pictured forgiveness — an orchard
carpeted with apples, bruised and fallen.

War Remnants Museum, Ho Chi Minh City

The bulk of the remnants are photographs
of crimes — a naked girl whose skin is on fire
from splotches of napalm, a vacant hillside
with dead trunks, relics of Agent Orange.

Larger remnants sit on the grounds outside —
an American Chinook aircraft,
a Russian-built tank, a fragment of sewer
from Thanh Phong in which three children hid.

Some remnants have sprung into being
since then — In carts and wheelchairs and braces
at the building's entrance, a chorus
of song-filled children, playing instruments

with toes and prostheses, living remnants
of hubris, as is the ingot of shame
in my heart. During the applause, they smile
at the audience and nod their heads.

Cesium 137

> In Goiania, Brazil, "an old radiotherapy
> source was taken from an abandoned
> hospital site...."

In a field scattered with axles, fenders,
sets of steel wheels, whole bodies of cars,
children discover the marvelous powder.
At twilight they return with their friends
to revel in its phosphorescence.

One child smears cesium on his arms
and climbs beneath an abandoned car
to augment his glow. His sister makes rouge
of the powder on her cheeks and tastes
the miraculous stuff. Others shove dabs
into their pockets and plastic purses.

This is the treasure they had hoped
to discover, the cairn of their small lives
burst open — beyond their parents' drab
existence, their loveliness aglow at last.

The children begin to die within the day
Heads smoldering, mucosa raw,
their bodies vacillate and weaken
hour by hour, consumed by innocence
and radiant desire.

Burial Rite

Vedbaek, Denmark, 5000 BCE

They decorated her dress with boar's teeth
and tiny shells, smeared her limbs with ochre,
and placed her head on a deerskin pillow.

They put the body of her newborn son
into the crook of her arm and covered him
with the soft, extended wing of a swan.

For protection on the perilous journey
to the land of the dead, they laid
a freshly-sculpted flint knife in her hand.

In her leather-like stomach, the remains
of a mother's last meal before giving birth —
seeds of wild plants. Some of them sprout.

Sacrament of the Sick

Limpopo, South Africa

What if Flora came back, not made of sticks
and sinews creeping across the room
on granny's arm, but in a bright blue robe
with shimmering yellow lines and a dozen
jangling bracelets, and the cardboard coverings
of her windows turned to glass, and the bent
aluminum fork her daughter is digging
in the dirt with became a doll dressed in glitter
and sequins. What if Flora could ambush
the Minister of Health at the point of a knife
and imprisoned her in an underground chamber,
where she would tie the Minister's tongue
and stick a tube in her throat and siphon out
the Minister's moisture, until she was dry
as a mummy from the Kalahari.
What if Flora came back, not struggling
toward her bed in muslin, but wearing
a brash Sotho blanket and crimson turban,
dancing *Morena boloka setjhaba.*
What if, after Benedict anointed her
with oil and chrism and made the sign
of the cross on her lips, Flora could pour
protein and lemon juice and garlic bits
into the Minister's throat until her skin
shimmered with life, and Flora forgave
her cruelty and lies. What if everything
was different, and Flora's daughter
didn't die, and Flora's husband
kept his pants buttoned. What if Benedict's
blessing ascended to God, like a comet
skidding from here to the Oort cloud.

Shall Inherit

Pale as clay they come to school
in Pineville, Kentucky,
carrying the cardboard cups
we gave them, as directed, full,
wrapped in newspapers and bags
with rubber bands in both directions.
They march to teacher's desk,
watching the wall of crayoned squirrels
instead of us and drop their cups.

The children — gaunt as parents are,
tight as vines, and bred from one
tough root — march barefoot
through these hills until they reach
the porch of Redbird Mission School
and put on shoes. The rat-tat-tat
of shoes on polished boards
wakes me to the work ahead —
spin and fix, stain the cysts.

I watch those sinewy children
with the sweet queerness of ether
in my mind, and hear formaldehyde's
weird voice say *Ascaris*
and innocence. One child has tapeworm,
one child has hook. With their small
serious eyes like coals, they come
on clay roads to Redbird Mission School
wearing the shrunken heads
of ancestors on their shoulders.

At the Egyptian Market in Istanbul

Pomegranates. Sacks of spice. Garish dolls
with battery-powered hips gyrate on a crate
covered with carpets. What infernal heat!

A folding table with an oversized jar.
In its murky water, hundreds of leeches,
clumps of them, cling to the greenish glass.

A somnolent man in a tent-like garment
sits beside the sign – ARTHRITIS (in English).
BLOOD CLOT. SWELLING. VARICOSE VEIN.

A small boy slips behind the table
and dips his hand into the leeches'
container. The vendor swears and swats him.

Leeches wave like kelp in a dirty tide.
The blood-sucking monsters thrive in the heat.
Gyrating belly dancers slow down and stop.

"Pair Chase Boy for His Urine"

Tucson Daily Courier
October 28, 1998

Five bucks to piss in a cup, no strings attached,
cries the man in the muscle shirt. He seems sincere.
Raunchy, but it's a solid plan he's hatched.

The woman with a dirty scarf. They're matched,
like two cracked cups. Nothing there to fear.
Five bucks to piss in a cup, no strings attached.

Just step behind the bushes — job dispatched.
The two of them are desperate to appear
squeaky clean. It's a solid plan they've hatched.

Lanky hair, sallow skin, their faces splotched
with hopefulness. I wonder if it's fair.
Five bucks to piss in a cup, no strings attached.

A dirty specimen — they'll both be scratched
from rehab in a snap. So much for their
second chance. It's a solid plan they've hatched.

Should I do it? Or should I stay detached
and tell the cops? Or just get out of here?
Five bucks to piss in a cup, no strings attached.
I'll ask for more. A solid plan they've hatched.

Montazah Gardens, Alexandria

On the corniche a brightly colored knot
of children begs an American woman
to repeat their names — Habibah, Neema,
Husani, Ife. Smiling pink scarves
push closer. An impish boy asks her,
Do you live in a mansion? Can I come
to New York? Behind them, the bay's
flat arms open, and on the horizon
sit scribbles of the distant city,
concealing its squalor and violence.

Among the orange and azure robes
and giggling girls, one wearing a niqab
stands a head taller than the others.
As I place a frame around these children,
much like the city frames the park and the park
its lovers, she raises her hands, palms out,
thumbs together, toward the camera,
as if to frame her invisible face —
or photograph me. Through the slit, the bridge
of her nose appears, her luminous eyes.

Night Vision

Uluru, Australia

Above the black desert
a bewilderment of pinpricks
shine. A pair of red twins.

Antares, a ball of gas
nearly the size
of the orbit of Jupiter.

The arid planet Mars,
a residue of rock
tortured by blasts of dust.

Boiling furnace, tiny speck.
One emits, one reflects.
Past progressive, present tense.

One's distance measured in time,
one's size in distance,
like my heart's attachments —

some stare, others twinkle.

Phone Call from Alaska

for Heather

That you were shot. That it was only a flesh wound
in your left upper arm. That it came through the window
above the sink in your basement apartment.
A pop. A pin. That you had no idea what it was until
a burn below your shoulder, glass shards in the sink.
Straight through your meat. It's nothing serious,
you insist. Again.

I have to imagine your teapot whistling.
Your oatmeal. Your pieces of peanut butter toast.
I have to imagine it all. Not a sniper,
but a kid getting a jump on Halloween morning.
A trick, but no treat. A scare, but no harm, you repeat
for the fifth time.

Twenty-two caliber. That they found the bullet
on the kitchen floor under the table near your boots.
That you drove to the ER, took the rest
of the day off work. That it was meaningless, random,
so to speak, you chuckled, shot in the dark,
but it made you think.

Dr. Barrone

The first time Doctor Barrone came
to my home, I lay on the sofa
drenched in fever, shivering with fear.
Barrone smelled like a monsignor
smoking a cigar. His nose and mustache
hovered maliciously above me
and sprayed. He poked at my stomach
He toyed with my ears. Just as his paws
were poised to tighten their grip around my neck,
Barrone pulled them back and burst
into his wicked leer. My mother,
God bless her, was convinced that he cared.
From a jar in his bag, he stuffed
a packet with the pills that turned my teeth
yellow, a remnant of that encounter
that still colors me. My mother
smothered the tablets in applesauce
and insisted I eat the poison,
until I picked up my pallet and walked.

The Biopsy Room: Prostate

Each punch of the device
thuds in my boggy brain
a fraction of a second
after its teeth bite
a sliver of prostate —
a miniature dragon
attacks my rectum,
a white-clad assistant
slips fragments of tissue
into labeled containers.
Twelve punches, a dozen
vicious bites, the twelve
great labors of Hercules,
especially his capture
of Cerberus, three-headed
sentry of the underworld,
the twelve apostles of Christ,
especially the last, Jude,
patron of impossible
causes, the twelve Knights
of Camelot, especially
Gawain, the purest of heart
who lopped off the head
of the Green Knight,
but found forgiveness,
the twelve Olympian gods,
especially Apollo,
my protector, the zodiac's
twelve constellations,
including Libra, which
augurs balance and grace —
The last punch reminds me
of Cancer, whose sharp pincers
won't let go.

Incomplete Knowledge

Pretending it didn't hurt, he got up
from his recliner and held out the film
he had badgered his doctor to give him.

By the dim lamp, the x-ray disclosed
a fuzzy coalescence where his left lung
should have been. And fluid on the right.

My father-in-law asked what I thought
of the situation, while commenting
in a casual voice that he had decided

on radiation, a plan the oncologist
had convinced him would be effective.
I stared at clusters of finger smudges

on the film's surface — they irked me.
His face, drained now that its padding
had disappeared, seemed spiritual.

His cigarette hand fluttered above
his breast pocket for a pack. I nodded.
Radiation, I said, *is the best choice.*

Retrospective

Forty years passed. His body replaced
its cells, with the exception of his heart's
persistent pump and the mushroom-like paste
of his brain. Only scattered synaptic charts
of his internship remain, etched in myelin,
a few of them deeply. Nonetheless, a dried
umbilical cord connects that powerful womb
to the aging man, across a gulf as wide
as imagination. He doubts there's a thread
to follow, a blockaded door to open,
or a fusty corridor down which to tread
to a solution: those he hurt, the woman
he killed with morphine, more than a few
he saved. His ally, hope, will have to do.

So Many Remedies:
A Selection of Chekhov Poems

Chekhov Attends the Greek School

Taganrog, 1868

At the beginners' class in Greek School
teacher's cassock stands beside my bench,
but I can't remember the verb. He twitches,
flecking a bit of dandruff from his beard.
His switch is less harsh than my father's hand,
but the snickering children are crueler.

As the son of a peasant, I don't impress
these Greeks, who hang out at the docks,
cracking their knuckles. I sit on the bench
with my battered chalkboard, stealing a peek
out the window — once caught, I must kneel
for the rest of the day as punishment.

It's always the same drill: mornings at school,
home at noon, help at the shop until late,
keep my mouth shut, while father, who bows
so deeply to the merchant Greeks he scrapes
his forehead, throttles mother at supper
for making the soup too salty.

On Sunday my father drags me to church
for early Mass. *To labor on the Lord's behalf
is never harmful.* When my voice rises
from the choir, his eyes ignite with pride,
while near the sanctuary screen, the Greeks
nearly choke on their cuds of holiness.

The Student

When the student went out at dawn
the weather was fresh, but upon
his return at sunset, shards of ice
had begun to form at the pond's edge.

The gawky student burned in the wind.
Didn't winter's grip, he inquired
of his absent friend, squeeze us harder
each year, like a government?

Two women lingered at a bonfire
near the river, widows who lived
mostly on cabbage from their garden.
The daughter's husband had crushed her

until her eyes had become vacant.
The mother had a curious smile
that rose in her throat. The student,
warming his hands at the fire, told them

of Peter, who was so frightened
when put to the test, he denied
his friend, not once, but three times.
On a frozen night, the boy whispered,

just like this. The old woman's face
collapsed, and her daughter's reddened
as if she were blessed with grace,
but at the same instant, pierced.

And Peter went out and wept.
The boy's mind's entrapment cleared —
he knew that he, the two widows,
and the apostle were one,

inexplicably one. As he climbed
the hill toward home, it seemed to him
a shaft from the collapsing sun
that slid across his face was warm.

148

Chekhov Reflects on Nikolai's Death
from Consumption

Not that I didn't love him —
but he was a mad dog
of a brother, a thorn in my side.

He'd disappear for months
with his concubine
and emerge on a raft of shit.

What did my brother ever promise
that bore fruit?

Two months at his bedside —
I wondered around his rooms at night
and shuffled my implements.

What was said, was said
a hundred times. What wasn't said
was closer than comfort.

I left at the moment
you would have left him
if you, too, had been there
in the face of the evidence.

When I returned, another brother said,
He died in my arms.
And my sister told me,
I emptied the chamber pot.

Chekhov Searches for Happiness

I walk through the meadow — my boots glisten
from the morning's rain — deep in this land
is a trace of the numinous.

A fragrance — the rain has released the fragrance
of grass — some days
I am detached like a stone out of place
but today my heart is enormous.

Today the meadow blazes with wormwood
and tiny bright flowers. Today I recall the tales
of incredible riches, of buried treasure.

Ghost-ridden peasants went to their graves
in search of a map, a key — *if only* was welded to their breasts,
a part of their lives,
what if I found it was their shadow, their bread.

What if I found it lives in me, too —
a monotonous cricket
in the moist steppe of my experience.
It blunts my ears, my soul.

What if I found it makes my attention move elsewhere —
when the cricket chirps
I am unable to feel the movements of my heart —
Today the cricket is silent.

Where will I search for the buried treasure? Where will I dig
for my casket of happiness?
I'll dig right here.

Six Prescriptions of Chekhov

1.

If you talk too much
the blood will rush to your lungs
and deprive the brain,
so don't chatter
and avoid getting constipated.

2.

If you are afraid of stressful living
turn yourself into a smelt or sturgeon.

If you don't want Russia to blow up like Sodom,
go to Kiev for the Easter procession.

If you are fed up with so much suffering,
potassium iodide is a splendid thing.

3.

The doctor I work with
is quiet and homely.
We nearly always disagree.
I give good tidings
where she imagines death
and when she prescribes a dose
I double it.

4.

Don't let her have porridge,
sunflower seeds, or bread.
If she asks for vodka,
give her a cigarette.

Don't improvise
unless you think about it.

5.

Some are for arrowroot.
Some are against.
Others have no strong feelings
either way.

As soon as the bowels become loose,
abandon it.

6.

I grow weary of peasant women
and tired of iodoform.
A girl with worms in her ear,
a monk with syphilis, an opinion
about the nature of illness,
the tedious powders. Phooey!

Oh, sweet sounds of poesy,
where are you?
Come, climb through my window.

On Sakhalin Island

When I entered the hut
and tried to speak to the boy
he winced with his shoulders
and backed away.

The hut smelled, the boy
was barefoot,
scrawny, sodden, and the rain
demonic.

When I asked about his father
he said, *I don't know my father.
I'm a bastard.*

I could hardly hear his voice
in the violent wind —
it drove wedges of rain
through kinks in the hut's walls.

The boy said his mother was sent
to Sakhalin Island
because of her husband.
My mother's a widow, he explained.

She killed him.

Empty Soup

We made a soup last week
from turnips and thistles —
that's how poor we've become.

In the mill, our machinery
is down — we sweep the floor
all week with politics.

Better to be a free man
than a cog — stories like this
are spice for our pot.

In our lives, too — the voice
of the Russian nation
is drab and heroic

like a long family trip
after a death — so much
to do, so little time.

Empty soup, that's what
the woman from Novotny
served for her supper.

Yes, I am grateful,
she said, even for the thistles
in the cracks of my life.

Cholera

Melikhovo, 1892

The epidemic bursts from Astrakhan
and roars north, pushing flames of panic
in front of it. They say the corpse's
muscles twitch for hours after death,
and peasants whisper the dead still speak.

Priests take to the road with their icons
pestering their saints for forgiveness.
A crowd of ruffians enters the room
we are storing the drugs in and smashes
the bottles. You wouldn't believe their stories.

They say doctors are causing the outbreak —
it's a scheme to keep the population down.
They say big government is behind
the conspiracy — we who work in the field
are dupes, the tools of perdition.

Cholera seems to strike for no reason —
it hits the vigorous, the young spill their guts.
The peasants place their bets on evil —
the doctors' or the czar's — as the source of it.
How can they face life if death is meaningless?

They run to the clinic, bludgeon the doors,
chase out the sick. *Escape from the death house!*
There is enough truth in their ignorance
to make you wonder, enough calamity
in their passion to deepen the burden.

The Hypnotist

He literally performed miracles...
some he paralyzed, others he had
balancing on chairs by their neck and heels.
                Anton Chekhov, "A Hypnotic Séance"

Fix your eyes on this shiny gem.
Follow it with your gaze
as it swings like a pendulum.

Avoid attention to your maze
of contradictions. Think of a saw's
back and forth, ripping your haze

of indecision. Imagine the wall
you've built around you — crashing.
Imagine the cataracts fall

from your eyes, the virulent rash
quiet and fade. Take those deep,
smooth breaths. Your determined dash

into the future, your uncertain past,
mean nothing if you have faith
that redemption will come at last.

Our audience yearns to believe.
There will be an ovation if only
you pay attention, as I relieve

all responsibility and doubt,
and grant you the liberty
to do exactly what you want.

Chekhov Makes Love at a Distance

Sweet marvelous actress,
I bow down before you,
so low that my forehead
scrapes the dry bottom
of the well in my heart —
as a result of your absence
this well is fifty-six feet deep.

My pigeon, you write me
what the weather is like
in Moscow, but I can read
the papers for weather.
My room and my bed
are like a summer cottage,
abandoned. Are not
both of us incomplete?
I'm weary without you.

My sweet dog, last page
of my life, I'm torn up
by the roots, but the body
won't move. I'm hoping
my health holds — you don't
need a seedy old
grandfather in your bed.
O, how I envy the rat
that lives beneath the floor
of your theater!

The Cherry Orchard

If a great many remedies
are suggested for some disease,
it means the disease is incurable.
        "The Cherry Orchard"

The end of the century
has come upon us
without a sign of release
or the beginning of justice.
We're selling the orchard
to pay our debts
and reminiscing about
love's excitements,
life's mistakes. I suspect
a century ago the hearts
of the people sitting here
were just as generous,
intense, and cruel as ours.

A miniature flower
thrives in the moisture
and dust of a broken
pavement — this is the gist
of the matter. We want
so strongly to believe
the flower will spread
everywhere. How quickly
it dies! If the disease
had a cure, we would not need
so many remedies.

For Oysters Only

Dear Anton, I have to tell you
the story of your deathbed at the spa
at Badenweiler is compelling — *Ich sterbe*,
you whisper in German. You struggle
to raise your desiccated body,
drink in one swoop a glass of champagne,
flash Olga a radiant smile, collapse
on your side, and softly breathe your last.

The perfect wisdom of your death
is too enticingly redemptive.
I have to force myself not to believe
in its romance. Instead, I try
to imagine how dopey with fatigue
the two Russian students are
when Olga pounds their door at midnight
and sends their diminishing footsteps
in search of a doctor. Instead, I try

to visualize your pale rags of lungs,
your fever raving about Japanese threats,
your soft words dissolving to gibberish,
the sound of a moth beating its wings
on an electric lamp. Instead of your
triumphant funeral, I call to mind
the train that carries your body to Moscow
in a boxcar labeled, *For Oysters Only*.

Previously Uncollected Poems

Journey

Sixteen blocks to the hospital from home
at 47th and Pine, sidewalks damp,
lighting dim — I imagine trekking a high pass
in Bhutan. Yaks clang. Prayer flags flutter
in the chill between rocks. No Chevy Impala
on concrete blocks near the intersection
of 44th and Spruce. No stench of dog turds
from a storm drain. I imagine Sarawak,
the rivers, their tributaries of doubt. Dawn frost
replaced by humid heat. A trick that involves
an imperceptible effort — my mind blocks
the reality of row houses, muffler shops,
and work. One voiceover breaks up, another
announces the arrival of 34th Street,
border of a broad savanna where wolves
of compassion roam. At 6 AM I enter their lair
and push my geographies into a drawer
beneath my skull, among cabinets containing
stacks of patterns, procedures, and my precious
thimblefuls of love. In this pack, I'm the adopted son.

The Elephant with a Cork in Its Butt

for Ken Rogers

The elephant fetish from Mozambique
with a cork in its butt
into which you empty your spirit of grief.
The wooden mortar and pestle
from Mindanao and the Navajo medicine belt
with bells stitched on it. After you died
I tossed them, along with stacks of files
and boxes of musty survey forms
forty years old. I dumped your stuff
from my drawer — an envelope with a note
about what I should do if you died
in surgery and the keys to your cabin
tied to a piece of pine you had carved
and finished. In addition, a three-inch
naked Chinese woman, a device
that permitted a patient to point
to the place it hurt without submitting
to examination. A boar-faced god
screwing an iron goddess, a cobra
wrapped around his shoulders. An icon
of the Virgin. A set of gourd rattles.
All that junk of hope, like the elephant
with a cork in its butt, a fetish
container into which you spill out
your spirit of grief.

Adelaide

Adelaide lies encased in ice,
a tiny fist without an arm,
and can't breathe on her own,

or keep her pressure up
and beat the odds
with broken chromosomes.

Three docs, a nurse, an aide
who soothes her, a chaplain
and a social worker

strung together for the climb
by glacial rope, a taut
compassion wraps their waists.

She's bled again, her brain
has dammed the fluid in.
Imagine an arctic waste

where climbers toss a rope
across a wide crevasse
that Adelaide cannot catch.

Death Benefits

We have a small burial allotment
set aside for cases like this
and a large American flag
you can pick up at the office
during working hours, or have sent
to your home, but not in time
for the funeral.

There is also a form to fill out
in case he was orphaned, or damaged
when young, or his mind
took a turn for the worse, but only
if the turn occurred during the war,
in which case your loved one
may also be entitled to something else.

Sometimes survivors ask questions
regarding what happened —
Did my loved one have pain in the end?
Could he have survived, if things
had gone differently? We suggest
you think twice before asking.
These questions won't bring him back.

In summary, we did everything we could.
We did even more than was expected.
We worked double shifts, often
without lunch, often half-sick ourselves.
No one has ever cared for a person
the way we cared for your loved one.
Please accept our sincerest regrets.

Pantoum on Sayings of William Osler

I propose to clarify the secret of life,
Sir William said, enjoying his joke.
The grace of humility is a precious gift.
Uncertainty generates hopes and fears.

Sir William insisted, enjoying his joke,
Cultivate, gentlemen, the art of detachment.
Amid fear of uncertainty, hope endures.
Apply obtuseness in judicious measure.

Cultivate, gentlemen, the art of detachment.
Adopt an exterior view from within
and apply obtuseness judiciously.
The past is with us, never to be escaped.

To adopt an external view from within
is necessary, but difficult to attain.
The inescapable past resides inside us.
Its gentle influence makes life worth living.

How necessary, but difficult, to attain
a steady foothold for our stricken souls —
the gentleness that makes life worth living.
The faculties upon which we all depend

pace unsteadily through our stricken souls,
bringing disappointment and sometimes failure.
The faculties upon which we all depend —
Oh, that I had the heart to spare you grief! —

disappoint us in the end, and my failure
to teach you the secret of life, make clear
my heart, and spare yours, may have caused grief.
The grace of humility is a precious gift.

Mother and Child, 1943

The baby is six weeks old. You carry him
to Texas in a basket in November.
The train crawls with raucous young troops
who bash you with stories, pinochle, beer.
And one pea-coated boy with a look
in his eye relinquishes his seat to you.

You sleep. No, first I see you watching
the backs of buildings out of Pittsburgh —
freight cars and sidings, barrels and crates.
The track keeps shooting out of sight
in front of the train, but all you can do
is watch sideward and smear the window's soot
with your handkerchief.

I never see the baby crying. Or feeding.
My only image is of you holding the child
beside a cold window between...
The window is always *between*. Between your dad
in Pittsburgh and the baby's in Texas.
Between you and the elderly woman
whose forgetfulness will one day betray you.
Between the baby and the child, the son, the man,
who looks back into the train at you.

Do you sleep? Or do you remain awake
and wonder what will happen? How can you know
the homesick sailors will pass your baby around
at dinner and put little gifts in his basket?
That it will start to snow, when it never snows
in Texas? That, after the war, your train
will keep on crawling down the Ohio Valley
on its way to Texas, night after night,
the same train, same trip, same basket,
with each of us trying to see the other
through that same black pane.

Home Repairs

for Benjamin

My son never laid his eyes
on window weights until tonight.
Tacks between his lips,
he mallets the sash into place,
with a sense of what is going on
with wood, prys and pulleys —
a knack I never had.

The cords were broken
when we bought the house.
He was six. His grandfather looked
at the shape of the windows, shook his head,
and offered to fix them. For a price,
my help. A price I refused to pay.

It took me ten years to crack this paint,
pull the sash and string the pulleys.
Now my son is finishing the job.
He taps in the tacks and steps back to look
like his grandfather would.

Black glass reflects a balding man,
shorter than his broad-shouldered son.
And a third figure between them —
he has not left us alone.
In this way, I begin to love him.

On Ice

Walking on the lake, my mother
makes a game of it. She crunches
a dozen steps beyond the beach
like an Eskimo hunter
while wind blows all the way
to Canada. My mother returns
with a joke about walking on water,
goes out on the ice and returns
a dozen times
until I put my arm
around the hump of her back
and lead her to the rumbling car
where my own children wait.

When my mother dies,
I see her walk
from the quay in Cleveland
toward the horizon
without turning back.
On that quiet day, I hear her feet
crunch
crunch
crunch
across the ice and disappear.

After a Photograph of Anne Holding
Her Morning Cup of Coffee

This moment teased by light from what is past
and fixed on paper here still has the feel
of waking; your coffee, to deal the last
telling blow at night and vaguely steal

a grip on day. Somehow your turban seems
a chrysalis for embryonic hair,
and your eyes, half-opened as they are, scheme
to steady cup and hand. The human care

to work out who you are is still asleep
with common sense, desire and even love.
Sitting there, you haven't tried to keep
within yourself or even tried to give.

In the rifled box I have of memory,
bulging with moments that may hold a clue
to what I am, it is a joy to see
this rose, a morning star, an orchid, you.

Satyagraha

> In June 1893, a young Indian lawyer
> was forcibly ejected from a 1ˢᵗ Class
> train in Pietermaritzburg, Natal.

1. The conductor

In a minute his anger at the Indian
subsides and he continues his rounds
in the First-Class carriages, making certain
Afrikaners sleep securely and sound.
A door clanks. The train jerks into motion
only a few minutes late, but even so
the image of that brash little man
in that three-penny suit sticks in his caw,
that brown stud snappy with cash, as if money
made a difference to God's eternal plan,
the European burden, the lonely
trek to perfection. He paces the train
in the dark. *Why did that fancy Indian
get me so riled up? Well, I taught him.*

2. The brash little man

Inside the Pietermaritzburg station,
the miniature lawyer defiantly looks
at his Johannesburg ticket, wondering
why has this happened? Neither books
nor experience had prepared him for this
desolate night. Edgy in his seat,
he leaps up straight, unable to resist
a burst of adrenalin. With restless feet
and blinking eyes, he realizes his train,
by Anglo fiat, must be Second Class
because of race. Must he endure the shame?
Or should he fight it? Accept this harass-
ment, or stand fast? *I shall not comply,*
decides Mohandas K. Gandhi.

Used Golf Balls

The road that circles Setauket Pond
passes an African Methodist
Episcopal Church, where the pastor
posted my favorite sign —
Used Golf Balls. 35 Cents.
They're Almost New. I wonder
how they redeem those balls?
I haven't played a round in forty years
but one of these days I'll buy a bucket
of used balls from the pastor's wife
and swat one over the wetlands
below the pond. I'll let a second go.
Swat. And another. *Swat.* I'll scatter
those selfish Canada geese to the wind.
Passion! Yes, I must change my life.

Theories of the Soul

Twenty Cases Suggestive of Reincarnation
by Ian Stevenson, 1918-2007

The soul I grew up on
begins at conception
bearing its ticket
to perdition or heaven.

A more plausible version
disintegrates at death
without a suggestion
of recurrence or wrath.

Your children remember
lives before this one,
traumatic encounters
in village and home.

Fanciful stories, but
unanswered questions.
Am I an old soul's
hundredth edition?

I look into my depths
to discover a mark
that I wasn't extinguished
but re-embarked,

neither gifted for goodness
nor exacted for shame
by an improbable wizard
behind the curtain.

174

The Talking Cure:
New Poems

Three Points of Reference

1.

A Visit to Polk Institute

It was natural for us to visit the idiots
at Polk Institute. Though abuzz
with curiosity, we took it slowly.
First, morons playing table-top games
in the solarium bustled around us,
smiling. Next, came the imbeciles'
oversized faces in chairs at the foot
of their beds. Last, a cavernous hall
of cribs with idiots in them, babies
big enough to thicken our skins
with truth, an important precaution
for doctoring. Nothing is more natural,
the idiots told us, than imperfection,
and nothing is more solemn than silence.
We were aliens with tanks on our backs
containing a gas that protected us
from human feeling. We knew nothing.

2.

Vivisection

A lab assistant injected a bolt
of anesthetic before we began
to cut, aping as well as we could
surgical steps from a book the dog
had never read. *Cannulate the heart*
was crucial to proving once again
that an increase in ventricular volume
enhances the force of contraction.
After we left the lab, an assistant
gave each dog a lethal shot to shorten
its suffering. At the time
a dog's death in the lab meant nothing.
Villages were dying in Vietnam.
Riots were breaking out across the land.
We were consuming bites of the fruit
of knowledge, confident in the track
that lay ahead. In an arrangement
with the pound, thirty mutts showed up
at the loading dock, and the innocent
soon-to-be-healers killed them.

3.

The Dying Psychiatrist

Dr. Frankl died after a placid week
in the hospital of something that hadn't
smothered his questioning. His bearded,
skeletal face would begin to enquire
about my life each day before I slipped
my stethoscope under the sheet
he kept pulled to his neck. A psychiatrist
expiring in a way that didn't require
I do much, yet work needed to be done
in other rooms. His strangely irrelevant
questions were awkward — Was I happy?
Did they treat me right? What did I like to do
when I left the hospital? In those days
I tended to sit for a minute or two
on the edge of a patient's bed
while completing my routine. When Dr. Frankl
reached for my hand and pressed it in his,
a movement that made me tighten,
his voice broke up, like a clod of dirt
in a dry riverbed. Days before he died,
I told him I was desperate to get away.

The Talking Cure

for David Pearson, MD

At eighty-one, my friend, who once was told
he'd never graduate in medicine
because his heart was tender, climbs the stairs
after seeing his last patient. For years
he's helped a retired lieutenant examine
the slippage of his inner knots by talking.

We sip iced tea. *They don't teach the talking*
treatment anymore. We used to be told
that words matter. Remember? He's examined
syllables and silence as his medicine
for decades. His cheeks ravaged by the years
on steroids, twitch with dampness, and he stares

at melting ice cubes. He recalls the stairs
to paradise — that's irony talking
through regret — and he's dissecting the years
with sharp New England wit. I never told
him of my weakness, but he knew. Has medicine
hardened his heart? I avoid examining

mine, not today, as we examine
the world through a kitchen window, and I stare
at Narragansett Bay, a medicine
just visible between the trees. Talking
rakes up leaves. What's beneath? Truth be told,
neither of us has ended where those years,

when youth seduced us, promised. Every year
accounted for, but when I examine
my conscience — an expression that tells
a lot about my childhood — what stares
at me is gratitude, not guilt. Talking
to my friend this afternoon is a medicine

that pares away scarred skin, a medicine
of acceptance — his fighting for years
to be heard, the ease with which I talked
a good game — all of which we examine
with astonishment. I descend the stairs
to the door as we continue talking

of medicine and our examined
routes, frenetic years, a world that stares
at pain without telling while we do the talking.

The Egyptian Goddess

I sneak a sandwich under my coat
and walk to the museum across the street,
where Sekhmet, the scorcher of multitudes,
glares from a granite throne. The ancient
Egyptians are often alone at midday,
except for a guard who sits beside the door
with a newspaper. My visits are short
and unpredictable, like chest pain, trauma,
stroke, and attempted suicide — each one
bumping against the other. I wear scrubs
to visit the mistress of terror,
whose impassive lion face and vacant eyes
ignore me. Sitting on a stone bench, I watch
as I eat lunch and ask the goddess,
Tell me what it means, moonlighting
as patroness of physicians, when
your day job is goddess of annihilation?
Is utter destruction a partner to healing?
While Sekhmet's blip-like granite breasts
are dry, I drink my fill from a thermos.
I ask her, Are you responsible
for the man they pulled from the Schuylkill River
this morning? For the explosion and burned
survivors? The cherisher of carnage
stares at the glass case of a sarcophagus
across the room. Do you create havoc
to set your physicians struggling in vain?
Divine mistress of suffering, explain.

Compassion

The temporoparietal junction
sets the pace and lets
the insula chime in, so brain
creates compassion out of nothing.

My right midcingulate gyrus
connects me to myself and others
by the honey of kindness
and the milk of empathy,

Behind the pools of beatitude
in which I frolic, are networks
of neural tracks, leafless shoots
on an aging tree behind my house —

If I spray them with a mist
of grace to nourish
and make them bloom, may I carry
their blossoms to heaven?

Reflection

I imagine my mother's dementia
began like this — occasional smudges,
blots, that gradually coalesced.

Incline suddenly fails to appear
when I want it. The percentage rise
on a treadmill, an old funicular,

hides behind a blot that wasn't there
earlier. I pester the blot's edges
by suggesting *diagonal, upwards,*

to no effect. When *incline* comes back,
I've taken the train to another
location. How many times was she blocked

before the sludge hardened? I once thought
subtractions swept her identity away
and left a shell, but now that I've begun

to forget on my own, I'm inclined
to believe my mother was silenced
by accretion, not loss, and she

survived as a blessed anchoress
bricked up in a cell between the walls
of a cathedral, looking out at us

through her peephole with tenderness,
as she awaited her salvation,
and we mourned her and withdrew.

Prison Break

I eavesdrop on the cells in your brain,
which are trying to bust out of a prison
surrounded by broken connections.

They make an almost inaudible hum
beneath mechanical whooshes and pings
surrounding your hospital bed. I listen

while sitting with your hand in mine,
not comforted by the confusion
of intensive care — I know your brain

is scheming, despite these machines
and my heartache, to escape. Its intention
is clear — get out while there is still time.

Some of the doctors say, *She's young and strong.*
Do the tunnelers in your brain hear them?
I eavesdrop — the messages you send are thin

and receding. There must be a billion
routes to escape your prison
and each one takes you away from me.

Shadow Children

These are children who don't have cancer,
who bunk overnight with their friends
while their siblings are getting another
immersion in poison, and their mothers
are napping beside beds in the hospital,
and their fathers have had to travel.

These are the children who try to diminish
their bodies, but unable to slip
into dying, or undermine blossoming,
or abandon desire, they discover
themselves at a loss about what to do next.

These are the children who excavate
tunnels in time and escape to the future,
whose bodies expand like buds and break off,
but cannot escape this difficult world
in which they don't become angels, and even
their innocence forgets what it was.

Cultural Exchange

He intends to amaze his visitor
with the guinea worm he's winding
from Mkale's matted abdomen
onto a dial stick, each day
a single rotation. And the scan
from the Cape — echinococcal cysts
blossoming in Dikobo's liver.

He's bought a tin of biscuits
for tea with the visitor,
whose diffident appearance
is disappointing. Regarding AIDS,
he intends to admit the Minister's
denial is crazy, but refrain
from political discussion.

The visitor lavishes praise
on Cuban advances
and dismisses his own nation's
excessiveness. This is curious,
but to be expected —
the American doctor has nothing
to lose. When the visitor asks

his opinion on how to improve
the hospital, fatigue radiates
from the Cuban's skin. He gestures
toward the worm, which he knows
will survive as an inclusion
deep within the visitor's brain.

Guardian Angel

Coronal section of the brain, lateral
ventricles, Vesalius, *De humani corporis
fabrica*, p. 609

The hole at the center of my brain
looks like angel's wings. My guardian
is lying on his belly looking down
through an open window at the base
of my skull. I imagine he keeps
a checklist. Heart. Pancreas. Lungs.
And so forth. When I was a child, he sat
on my shoulder and whispered advice
about resisting temptation. He was weak,
though, and soft-spoken. Much of the time
I didn't pay attention to his prodding.
He faded like a watercolor scene
in bright sun. Flew home to a Renaissance
altarpiece, where less was expected
of angels, and I was left to defend
my own virtue. I believe he is back now,
lying prone at the center of my brain.

I might be making too much of the gap
in the image. It's a wing-shaped sac
of fluid, my book says, positioned
to refresh the cells and drain their bilge,
a system of plumbing. The sac's shape
is coincidence. But I'm remembering
my guardian angel, and it looks like him
peering down, a cat on a windowsill
recording what's going on — Oxytocin,
dopamine, testosterone. And saying
nothing. It was comforting to be part
of a scheme, with a guardian angel,
inept though he was, assigned to me
to whisper advice. Anonymous now,
he listens, observes, and is eerily
detached. He could be anyone's angel.

Burial Mounds

I

Marietta, Ohio

Putnam and his people built their town
on the west bank of the Muskingum
beside an earthen causeway that led

a mile to a mound in the undergrowth,
its sides encased by thorny ligaments,
its ramp eroded, an impossible

apparition, a nearly perfect cone.
They said Phoenicians must have built it,
or one of the lost tribes of Israel.

Red savages could not have created
such perfection. Settlers scavenged
earthworks for clay and baked it to bricks.

They built a town from tissues of the past
and established a proscenium
on which they enacted their layers of life

atop a stratum of two thousand years.
A broken set of concrete steps
leads to the mound's top, where I view

the community of bones, a graveyard
sodden with fallen leaves — Adena,
Hopewell, Shawnee, and European.

II

Moundsville, West Virginia

A pickup creeps through scuds of old snow
and parks beside the vacant face of West
Virginia State Penitentiary. Ten below.

A thud of boots. The driver hoists herself
to the bed of her truck. Buds in her ears,
waving her red jacket above her head,

she dances — a jig, a clomp, an erratic
tattoo, producing cumulous clouds
from her mouth. Jeans and a sweater,

her arms slice the air. My parka zipped,
I climb to the top of Cave Creek Mound
across the street. The burial chamber,

an empty tomb, timbers collapsed,
has long since released its occupant.
I am not Peter, not Magdalene.

The woman dances a dance of her own.
A blessing? Or a curse on the prison
that sits where the chieftain buried here

with garlands of flowers and a conch
from the coast of Florida passed
from one mysterious land to another?

III

Chillicothe, Ohio

How very little they left behind —
ear plugs, pendants, and pottery
in a small museum. Not much to go on.

For hundreds of years they examined
events and had visions. Copper raven,
feathered spirit, pipe of the world above.

A grassy field exempt from this world
and set aside, remnants of earthworks
and mounds, encouraging tourists

enroute, like us, to a different place.
It could be a golf course, the mounds worn
to submission, a dozen captions describing

what used to be here. My childhood image
of Mound City — I press it between leaves
of this journey like a dried carnation.

How flimsy the evidence! If only
I could leave behind me a brilliant past,
a marker to extol my deeds —

I share the builders' twenty thousand genes.

Darwin's Prayer

He saw Darwin on his knees, and there
was no difference between prayer and
pulling a worm from the grass.
        Roger McDonald, *Mr. Darwin's Shooter*

Bright bunches
of gardenias
bloom in November,

the loam at their feet
moistened by dew
and spongy with debris.

As I fill my container
with handfuls of earth
alive with these

marvelous worms,
perfected in being
by the wisdom

of randomness,
I'm astonished
by gratitude.

Garden of Endurance

Cassia grandis, Costa Rica

Cassia fruit covers the forest floor,
a blanket of black sausage stinking
in the heat as it decomposes,
a mote in the eye of permanence.

Built for grinding by gigantic teeth,
Cassia's fibrous case condemns its seeds
to suffering, with neither mastodon
nor megatherium alive to free them

and distribute their undigested life
in mounds of shit. Its glory left behind
by climate, tooth, and claw, *Cassia*
endures by the grace of rodents

that gnaw its weakest fibers
and let a few fertile seeds escape
before they rot. Anachronistic
fruit, your survival — sweet tickle

of a breeze, illusion of peace,
diminishment that overcomes
extinction — is an inheritance
for my kind, too. A hopeful omen.

The Hippos of Camden, New Jersey

Having been rescued from life's burdens,
one of them gnaws the concrete barrier
at the edge of her enclosure.
Her huge snout toys with moist shards,
pushing them here and there
across the floor, her barrel-like behind
welcoming the audience.
Underwater, the other is motionless
for minutes. A child asks, *Is it dead?*
His mother is frantic for the beast
to begin breathing. He's utterly still.
When the beast's bleary-eyed snout
breaks into the open and snorts,
I, too, am relieved. The first hippo
glides into an artificial pool,
neither muddy nor exuberant
with being, not like the Zambezi River
with hundreds of huge hairless creatures
of her tribe. When a child tosses a piece
of popcorn into their enclosure,
do the hippos imagine
a tiny terrified frog? Their great yawps
expose useless tusks as big as fists.

The War of All Against All

Rapa Nui

Here on the island, where grassy flanks
of volcanos flow to the coast, they roped
the guardians' necks and tumbled them
to rubble. Each clan, driven by anger
and hunger, demolished the guardians
of others. Every one of them succumbed.

The ancestors had arrived in paradise
with taro, chickens, pigs, and ritual.
They gloried in finding a land so safe,
so abundant, and carved hundreds of moa
to protect it. With backs to the sea,
these gods of safe haven peered inward.

When descendants rolled the final giants
on beds of trunks from the last remaining
patch of forest, or toggled them back
and forth across eroded slopes and gullies,
the only columns of shade they had left
in piecing sun were sullen guardians.

Here on the island, a small girl, her chin
firm beneath full cheeks, sits on a rock,
selling six and eight inch moas to tourists.
Nine hundred giant faces. In all this rubble,
scientists were able to find only a single
obsidian pupil. One eye, and hundreds blind.

The Conference of Germs

In time the bacteria will convene
a conference to consolidate their plans
for coping with the loss of humans.

Those who colonized the humans
will be welcomed with respect and given
appropriate support, acknowledging

it was not their fault. The germs who live
in volcanic cracks will offer workshops
on the simple life. Others, on fixing

nitrogen. The more scholarly germs
will tackle the history of devastation;
specifically, the ingenious methods

humans used to eradicate their species.
Poet germs will sing of humans snipping
wisdom from their reproductive strands.

The principal theme will be the future.
Every germ will vow to continue
molding the planet, as duty demands.

The Persistence of Metaphor

Illness is not a metaphor... the most truthful way
of regarding illness is one most purified of...
metaphoric thinking.
Susan Sontag

I scrub my illness with disinfectant
to remove its horns and cloven feet.

I ridicule the crazy tales that pain tells,
sterilize them with ethylene oxide.

I freeze-dry a generous specimen
to rid my illness of implication.

Surely by now the magic must be gone.
Yet under my scope, a viable cyst

appears, containing a tiny body,
hands tied behind his back, a noose

around the neck, a prisoner
of narrative, wearing a grimace,

that begs for release.

Ghazal: Embodied

What happened to the *jinn* in my body
that ignited it? Now, I feel like nobody.

How clever to pluck the strings of animation,
fingers tightly crossed behind your body!

Let's face it. Shapeshifting is hardly a notion
that makes sense without consulting your body.

There must be a name for my aspiration,
something more elegant than *a younger body*.

Aloe vera serves as the basis for a lotion
that soothes the rash impertinence of body.

Looking between the sheets in fascination,
I seek the marvelous *jinn* of my body.

Goodness is good for you. That's an evasion
I can accept — but what about my body?

As the dervish spins, the vertiginous motion
whips him to the brink of being nobody.

Why insist on the elegance of creation
if you have toenails at the end of your body?

A kiss? A ritual? The cause of my elation
isn't for you to know. It's my body.

Automotive

I must have a fault in my timing belt
or a crack in the shaft assembly.

What do I know about ingredients
leaking from my tank? I've come to a stop,

stalled in the parking lot, burdened by
ignorance of what that's about.

My doctor's an antonym. She says
second gear, but I hear *reverse.*

A good mechanic, but innocent,
she lacks specs for my spark plugs

and data for my model year.
My doctor offers me a can of polish

and stiffens my wipers with advice.
She fixes leaks in two of my bald tires.

The Old Dilemma

The dilemma of the drowning child
occurs near the end of the chapter
on duties. He's terrified and can't swim.
You're the only person on a path
beside the shore. Just seconds to decide.
Jump to his rescue, or continue
on your way, after making the call
to 911? The chapter makes it clear
you're not wrong to avoid the risk
of hypothermia — the dilemma
always occurs in winter. Finding a branch
to reach out to his flailing hand
is virtuous, but not required. Consider
muck in your shoes and thorny bushes.
The blade of ethics rips close to your skin.
A voice from the underbrush murmurs,
dive in, dive in. But remember you're not
a saint. Ask, Why did the boy jump?
Think, Maybe his mother is on her way.
Or, Shouldn't he have learned to swim?

In Praise of Virtue

A student twitches in her seat,
irked at my wasting her time.
Fidelity, fortitude, compassion —
what a moldy scent they exude!
She wants content, words cut
from a block of granite, words
built with bricks from the ground up,
not old sheets waving in the wind.
Virtue! No wonder she Googles
an alternate route. Virtue, for her
is either fraudulent, or a track
too deep in the thalamus
to count. Pixel by pixel,
my student fades. *Wait! Wait!*

I'll juggle seven words at once
while walking on stilts.
I'll twist my face into a clown's
to capture her attention,
make her giggle with delight —
too late. Only a wisp
of her remains. I wanted to warn her
words can grind and abrade.
I wanted to show her the bruises.

Banana Harvest

Elderslie, Jamaica, 1968

I load my plate with ackee, salt fish,
chicken and yam, and accept a cup
of thick goat's blood and curdled milk.
Two trucks stacked with bananas sit
with their tarps flapping and glistening.
In the open pavilion, wind lashes
spurts of rain. Small pigs and a peahen
forage for scraps in a forest of legs.
Miraculous! The minister calls,
Praise God for all this plenitude!

Plenitude tumbles through my skull
like a stone nudged into the life
of a brisk stream. Heavy, but helpless
in flood. Mossy, but moving at last.
So many bunches. So generous
the mud. Such bosoms of plenty.
Taste and see the goodness of the Lord!
I have no more awkwardness to hide.
Neither image of the goat, nor burden
of the straight, to carry on my back.
I stand and sip that thick pink drink.

The Violin

A stringless violin
hangs on the wall
of my bedroom —
the crudely cut
unvarnished box
an artifact of the last
shimmering days
before my grandfather's
fingers lost
their keenness,
his eyes their sight.

The older brothers
commandeered
my grandfather's
Knights of Columbus
sword and his
oaken shillelagh
but left the youngest
a useless instrument.

Now that I'm old
I imagine the violin
has silent music
stored within, a cadence
of its own
that I might set free —
my grandfather's blessing
on his youngest son
whose son
now blesses them.

Knik Glacier

After a day scouring for blackberries in spitting rain
and gathering stones from the river, we sit around the fire
at midnight, an hour that would have been bright,
if not for the pewter cloud.

Nothing behind us moves. Ahead, the pier sloshes,
a stub of wavering boards on the glacial lake,
a forest of blackness beyond.

As I toss another gnarl of driftwood under the grate,
night's throat explodes with a shattering cough
as a mass of ice collapses into the lake, the glacier
calving, giving birth.

The jet-boat that brought us yesterday is back at the lodge.
The children are asleep in sweaters and jackets,
engaging in transformation.

Constellations

Great Bear and Orion — the two
I could distinguish as a child,
despite my grandfather's finger
pointing to others and, later,
the diagrams. A constellation
of symptoms was easier to see.

The first appeared in my body
like a splash of colorful pins
connected by lines. A red flush
under my eyes, the aching joints,
and sensitivity to sun — I ran
to my professor with lupus.

Later, I suffered a two-week
invasion of cancer. The omens
were plentiful. The lion, the fox,
the crab, and the dragon arose
from within, especially at night.
I monitored my heart rate

until experience grew tired
of reading signs that flickered
for a time, then one by one
disappeared in my obscure
interior, extinguished before
they queued to tell a story.

Great Bear and Orion remain
the only two I can trace. Time
hasn't helped me interpret
the stars, but I sense before long
a new constellation will form,
one I'll clearly discern.

Regarding Kindness

for John Wright

Still failing to put kindness
ahead of righteousness,
says an old friend, taking
a kilogram of blame
for condemning a child's
reckless decision. Fallen
from his narrow beam
of grace, my friend feels
empty, at a loss.

I remember the click-click
of my father's walker
approaching the kitchen
and my neck stiffening
in anger. He stood
at the doorway,
craning his puffy eyes
for company.

If I had wrapped my arms
around his chest...

When my grandson wraps his arms
around my waist
an envelope appears
in my rusty mailbox.

Acknowledgments

Special thanks to Patti Tana for her invaluable help in preparing the manuscript of this book. These poems, or earlier versions of them, appeared first in the following magazines:

Annals of Internal Medicine, "Astonishment," "Automotive," "The Conference of Germs," "Constellations," "Cultural Exchange," "Detached Concern," "The Biopsy Room: Prostate," "The Egyptian Goddess," "Empty Soup," "First Blood," "He Lectures at the Heritage Association Dinner," "He Lectures on Grace," "I'm Gonna Slap Those Doctors," "Interned," "The Man with Stars Inside," "Midnight Supper," "Ockham's Razor," "The Old Dilemma," "Prison Break," "Reflection," "Regarding Kindness," "The Secret of the Care," "The Shoe," "That Intern Dream," "The Talking Cure," and "War Remnants Museum, Ho Chi Minh City"

Bellevue Literary Review, "Reverence for Life" and "Theology"

Birmingham Review, "Poem for David"

Canadian Medical Association Journal, "The Poor Historian" and "William Carlos Williams Circumcises Hemingway's First Son"

The Cape Rock, "Guam"

Centennial Review, "Lima Bean"

Cumberland Poetry Review, "Don't Be Afraid, Gringo"

Embers, "St. Ronan's Finger"

The Examined Life, "Corrigan and the Giant"

Freshwater, "The Elephant with a Cork in Its Butt"

Great River Review, "My Father Sends Me Out for Tobacco"

Greenfield Review, "Mother and Child," "Jerusalem," and "The Dust of the West"

Journal of the American Medical Association (JAMA), "The Act of Love," "Adelaide," "Anita and Vladimir," "Cesium 137," "The Cherry Orchard," "Cholera," "Complications," "Cosmic Sonnets," "D-Day," "Deep Structures," "The Dying Psychiatrist," "The Exterior Palace," "The Garden of Endurance," "Happiness," "The Hypnotist," "Incomplete Knowledge," "Journey," "Keeping Dry," "Lachrymae Rerum," "Levitation," "McGonigle's Foot," "Metamorphosis," "My Machine," "My Uganda," "Pantoum on Sayings of William Osler," "The Persistence of Metaphor," "Ralph Angelo Attends the Barbeque," "Sacrament of the Sick," "Shadow Children," "Sirens," "Six Prescriptions of Chekhov,"

"Soundings: Three for the Stethoscope," "Take Off Your Clothes,"
"Tumbleweed," "A Theory of Labor," and "The War of All Against
All"

The Journal of Family Practice, "Brain Fever" and "First Photographs of
Heaven"

The Journal (Ohio State University), "Appetite"

Kansas Quarterly, "Banana Bread" and "Bursting with Danger and
Music"

The Lancet, "Body Count," "Chekhov Makes Love at a Distance,"
"Darwin's Answer," "Isn't," "The Pounds of Flesh," and "The
Student"

Literature and Medicine, "Alabama"

Manhattan Poetry Review, "Labrador" and "The Knitted Glove"

Negative Capability, "These Shards Are Wrist Bones"

North Atlantic Review, "Sunsets"

Old Red Kimono, "The Man with a Hole in His Face"

Oxford Magazine, "Good News"

Oyez Review, "Delicate Procedures"

Parting Gifts, "To the Mummy of a Thief in the Crypt of St. Michan's,
Dublin"

Patterson Literary Review, "Used Golf Balls"

The Pharos, "Virginia Ham" and "Forbidden Perfume"

Poetry East, "Levitation"

Prairie Schooner, "The Six Hundred Pound Man"

Pulse, "Retrospective"

Rattle, "The Origin of Light"

St. Andrews Review, "Chrysler for Sale"

South Coast Poetry Journal, "All Souls' Day," "Shall Inherit," "On Ice,"
and "Home Repairs"

Ulitarra (Australia), "Darwin's Barnacles"

Wordsmith, "Poison"

Zone 3, "Finches"

Poems reprinted in anthologies and other books:

"The Knitted Glove" and "Good News" in Reynolds R, Stone J. (eds.) *On Doctoring*, New York, Simon and Schuster, 1991, 1996, 2001.

"The Six Hundred Pound Man," "Skinwalkers," "The Man with Stars Inside Him," and "Medicine Stone" in Walker S, Roffman R. (eds) *Life on the Line: Selections on Words and Healing*, Mobile, AL, Negative Capability Press, 1992.

"Alabama" in Mukand J. (ed) *Articulations: Contemporary Poetry About Medicine*. University of Iowa Press, 1995.

"Complications" in Fox J. *Finding What You Didn't Lose. Expressing Your Truth and Creativity Through Poem-Making*. G. P. Putnam's Sons, 1995.

"I'm Gonna Slap Those Doctors" and "The Knitted Glove" in Wedding D. (ed.) *Behavior and Medicine* (2nd Edition), New York, Mosby, 1995.

"The Knitted Glove" in Carson RA. Beyond Respect to Recognition and Due Regard, in Toombs SK, Barnard D, Carson RA. (eds.) *Chronic Illness: From Experience to Policy*, Indiana University Press, 1995.

"The Six Hundred Pound Man" in Donley C, Buckley S. (eds.) *The Tyranny of the Normal*. Kent State University Press, 1996.

"Adelaide," "My Uganda," and "Lachrymae Rerun" in Breedlove C. (ed.) *Uncharted Lines. Poems from the Journal of the American Medical Association*. Albany, California, Boaz Publishing, 1998.

"The Shoe" and "Empty Soup" in LaCombe M. (ed.) *On Being a Doctor 2*, American College of Physicians, Philadelphia, 1999.

"Jerusalem" and "Poison" in Dittrich LR. (ed.) *Ten Years of Medicine and the Arts. 100 Selections from Academic Medicine)* Washington DC, Association of American Medical Colleges, 2001.

"The Old Man with Stars Inside" in Coles R, Testa R (eds.) *A Life in Medicine. A Literary Anthology*. New York, The New Press, 2002.

"The Six Hundred Pound Man" in Jarrell D, Sukrungruang I. (eds.) *What Are You Looking At? The First Fat Fiction Anthology*. New York, Harcourt, 2003, p. 152.

"The Old Man with Stars Inside" in Carlton R, Adler A (eds.) *Principles of Radiographic Imaging. An Art and a Science*, 4th edition, Clifton Park NY, Thomson Delmar Learning, 2005.

"Lachrymae Rerun," "Appetite," and "The Six Hundred Pound Man" in Moran D (Ed.), *The Light of City and Sea: An Anthology of Suffolk County Poetry*. Sound Beach, Street Press, 2006.

"Anatomy Lesson" and "Lachrymae Rerun" in *Pitt Medicine*, 2007/8, Winter.

"Death Benefits" in LaCombe M, Hartman TV (eds.) *Whatever Houses We May Visit: Poems That Have Inspired Physicians.* Philadelphia, American College of Physicians, 2008.

"The Rule of Thirds," in Doyle CT. *Healing Hands From the Cradle to the Grave. An Anthology of Medical Poetry*, Cork, Ireland, Litho Press, 2011, p. 83. Medical Poetry, Cork, Ireland, Litho Press, 2011,

"All Souls' Day" in Laine C, LaCombe MA (eds.) *On Being a Doctor*, Volume 4, Philadelphia, American College of Physicians, 2014.

About the Author

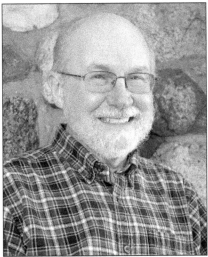

Photo by John Renner

Jack Coulehan is an Emeritus Professor of Medicine and Preventive Medicine, and former director of the Center for Medical Humanities, Compassionate Care, and Bioethics at Stony Brook University. His work in the medical literature ranges from clinical trials of depression treatment in primary care and studies of heart disease among Navajo Indians to essays on medical ethics, education, and humanities. His award-winning textbook, *The Medical Interview: Mastering Skills for Clinical Practice* (F. A. Davis, 5th edition, 2006) is widely used in American medical schools.

Jack's poems have appeared in literary magazines and medical journals in the United States, England, Ireland, Canada, and Australia; and his work is frequently anthologized. He is the author of six collections of poetry, including *The Wound Dresser* (JB Stillwater, 2016), which was a finalist for the 2016 Dorset Poetry Prize. Jack co-edited *Blood & Bone* and *Primary Care: More Poems by Physicians* (University of Iowa Press, 1998 and 2006) and edited *Chekhov's Doctors, a collection of Anton Chekhov's medical tales* (Kent State University Press, 2003). He previously published *Bursting with Danger and Music* with Plain View Press (2012).

Among Jack's honors are the Humanities Award of the American Academy of Hospice and Palliative Medicine and the Nicholas Davies Scholar Award of the American College of Physicians for "outstanding lifetime contributions to humanism in medicine." Jack currently serves as president of the Walt Whitman Birthplace Association.

Books by Jack Coulehan

The Wound Dresser — by Jack Coulehan (JB Stillwater Publishing Company, 2016)

Bursting with Danger and Music — by Jack Coulehan (Plain View Press, 2012)

Primary Care: More Poems by Physicians — edited by Angela Belli and Jack Coulehan (University Of Iowa Press, 2006)

The Medical Interview. Mastering Skills for Clinical Practice — by John L. Coulehan and Marian R. Block (F.A. Davis Company, edition 5, 2006)

Chekhov's Doctors: A Collection Of Chekhov's Medical Tales — edited by Jack Coulehan (The Kent State University Press, 2003)

Medicine Stone — by Jack Coulehan (Daniel & Daniel Pub, 2002)

The Heavenly Ladder — by Jack Coulehan (Ginninderra Press, 2001)

Blood and Bone: Poems by Physicians — edited by Angela Belli and Jack Coulehan (University Of Iowa Press, 1998)

First Photographs Of Heaven — by Jack Coulehan (Nightshade Press, 1994)

The Knitted Glove — by Jack Coulehan (Nightshade Press; 1991)

CPSIA information can be obtained
at www.ICGtesting.com
Printed in the USA
JSHW022230180520
5762JS00002B/4